CHOLESTEROL CLARITY

WHAT THE HDL IS WRONG WITH MY NUMBERS?

Jimmy Moore
with Eric C. Westman, MD

Victory Belt Publishing Inc.
Las Vegas

This book is dedicated to the memory of my late brother, Kevin Lee Moore, who needlessly died from heart disease and morbid obesity at just forty-one years of age because he was given all the wrong information about cholesterol and health.

First Published in 2013 by Victory Belt Publishing Inc.

ISBN 13: 978-1-936608-38-6

Printed in the USA

QC0519

Important Medical Disclaimer for *Cholesterol Clarity*

Jimmy Moore and Dr. Eric Westman (hereafter referred to as the "Authors") are providing *Cholesterol Clarity* (hereafter referred to as the "Book") and its contents on an "as is" basis and make no representations or warranties of any kind with respect to this Book or its contents. The Authors disclaim all such representations and warranties, including, for example, warranties of merchantability and fitness for a particular purpose. In addition, The Authors do not represent or warrant that the information accessible via this Book is complete or current.

The statements made about products and services have not been evaluated by the U.S. Food and Drug Administration. They are not intended to diagnose, treat, cure, or prevent any condition or disease. Please consult with your own physician or healthcare specialist regarding the suggestions and recommendations made in this Book.

Except as specifically stated in this Book, neither the authors, contributors, nor other representatives will be liable for damages arising out of or in connection with the use of this Book. This is a comprehensive limitation of liability that applies to all damages of any kind, including (without limitation) compensatory damages; direct, indirect, or consequential damages; loss of income, or profit; loss of or damage to property; and claims of third parties.

This Book provides content related to topics about nutrition and health. As such, use of this Book implies your acceptance of the terms described herein.

You understand that a private citizen, without any professional training in the medical, health, or nutritional field, coauthored this Book. You understand that this Book is provided to you without a health examination and without prior discussion of your health condition. You understand that

Contents

How to Use This Book

Most people who get a book tend to read it from beginning to end. We certainly encourage you to do that. There is a wealth of information contained in these pages, laying out the truth about cholesterol in easy-to-read language anyone can understand.

But this book is also meant to be a quick and practical guide for anyone who is getting cholesterol test results from their doctor. If, for example, some of your numbers seem to be out of normal range, your doctor may suggest taking medications as your first treatment option. Before you make that decision, we suggest you use this book as a research tool. Simply turn to the section that pertains to the number or numbers in question and there will be information regarding where you need to be for optimal health. In addition, we will tell you what you can do nutritionally and in your lifestyle to make improvements without necessarily turning to medications.

We have made every effort to figure out what the HDL is wrong with your numbers.

Introduction

Ever get the feeling there's a whole lot more to the cholesterol story than we've been told? For years, popular wisdom has held that having elevated levels of cholesterol in your blood is extremely dangerous, leading to heart attack, stroke, even death. Therefore, it must be lowered by any means necessary. Those means include cutting saturated fat and cholesterol from your diet and taking cholesterol-lowering prescription drugs. Sound familiar? Well, some of us took the time to stop and ask a few simple questions: Isn't the human body a lot more complex than this simplistic solution implies? Isn't our heath dependent on more than one single marker, like total cholesterol? And how and why did cholesterol become the villain? My name is Jimmy Moore and these are the big questions that I will answer for you in this book.

In the midst of writing *Cholesterol Clarity,* I paid a visit to my local Sam's Club, which offers its customers some free, basic health tests a few times a year. This is always an eye-opening experience for me, but not for the reasons you might think. I've been a keen observer of my health for the past decade, and in that time I've become fascinated by what is commonly defined by our culture as "healthy." The perfect example: my visit to Sam's Club.

I was there to get my total cholesterol and other health markers checked since they were offering these tests for free. As I was waiting in line, I happened to overhear the results for the young woman in front of me. She had a body-fat percentage of 39.7, which is considered very high ("normal" for a woman is 25–35 percent), as well as incredibly high blood pressure—something like 180/120 (healthy blood pressure is 120/80). But when her fasting blood sugar came back at 85 (in the 80s is ideal) and total cholesterol at 140 (anything under 200 is considered a "healthy" level), the nurse cheerfully exclaimed, "Wow! You are so healthy. Your cholesterol is under 200." The young woman said she had naturally low cholesterol, to which the nurse enthusiastically replied, "Yes, the less of that stuff [cholesterol] you have in your body, the better." All I could think was O…M…G!

Then it was my turn. The nurse and I chatted as I waited for my own blood work results. She commented on how healthy and vibrant I looked, and predicted that my numbers would be great. But all her enthusiasm quickly vanished, however, the moment the shocking results popped up on her screen. My total cholesterol came in at 322—widely considered exceedingly high by mainstream medical standards. She looked like someone whose dog had just been hit by a truck. Her tone became hushed and she nervously asked: "A-a-are you feeling okay?" I told her that I felt fantastic. But I don't think she believed me. She then asked what I was doing about my cholesterol problem. I explained to her that I wasn't worried about my cholesterol. "Oh, but you must take a medication to bring those unhealthy levels down," she responded. I told her that, in my opinion, cholesterol-lowering medications like statins are more harmful than helpful. After a few seconds of awkward silence, she nervously wished me well and sent me on my merry way, probably figuring I'd drop dead in the parking lot.

Health Has Been Reduced to a Numbers Game

My Sam's Club scenario is, unfortunately, not all that uncommon. When it comes to the medical profession, *high cholesterol* automatically means "poor health." And yet, one minute that nurse was telling me how great I looked; the next, after my numbers came in, she was assuming the worst. It's reactions like hers that prompted me to write this book, to help educate not only everyday people like you and me, but even those in the health profession who insist on promoting decades-old fallacies about cholesterol.

We live in the most technologically advanced period in history, with instant access to information on virtually any topic, including health. Type a keyword into a search engine like Bing or Google, and you'll get links to multiple sites purporting to know the answer to your question. It's a wealth of advice at your fingertips. But there's a big downside to "Dr. Google": the question of reliability. Who are the sources of the information? Can you trust them? Are they biased in any way? Is the information based on solid scientific evidence? These are critical questions when the subject is your health.

There's a lot of information about cholesterol out there—online, in magazines and newspapers, on TV—and all from so-called "experts." Most of it is contradictory or confusing or even outright false. How can you make informed decisions about what your own cholesterol test results mean if the messages are mixed? My hope is that this book will lift the clouds from your own good judgment, so that you, too, can begin to take control of your own health.

Who Is Jimmy Moore and Why Did He Decide to Write This Book?

In January 2004, my health was in shambles. I was thirty-two years old and my weight had ballooned up to 410 pounds; I was wearing 5XL shirts and sixty-two-inch-waist pants, and even those seemed to rip every time I sat down. I was dependent on three prescription medications—for breathing issues, high blood pressure, and high cholesterol. I had already watched my older brother Kevin struggle with morbid obesity; he lived through a horrifying series of heart attacks in 1999 when he was thirty-two. (Kevin eventually died from heart disease, diabetes, and obesity in 2008, at the age of forty-one.) Given all that happened to my brother, it's probably no surprise that I was motivated to do something about my own weight and health issues. I've learned a lot since then, and this book is my way of sharing some of that knowledge with those who have been misled.

I'll get into more specifics about my weight loss and health transformation story in my next book, *Keto Clarity*. But, briefly, I went on to lose 180 pounds in 2004 and weaned myself off the three "health-managing" drugs prescribed by my doctor. After just a few months of weight loss, the wheezing stopped; in less than six months my blood pressure was normal; after nine months, my cholesterol was low enough that I could come off the statin drugs. It was, both literally and philosophically, a transformative experience to say the least.

In 2005, I started writing a blog called *Livin' La Vida Low-Carb*. My intention was to educate, encourage, and inspire anyone else who might be dealing with a severe weight problem and the predictable health problems that come with it. My personal education skyrocketed a year later, when I became the host of the iTunes podcast *The Livin' La Vida Low-Carb Show with Jimmy Moore*. Through this top-rated Internet health radio show I have interviewed hundreds of the biggest names in the world of nutrition, medicine, research, and more. My natural curiosity and desire to soak up every bit of health-related information I came across made up for my lack of experience as a broadcaster and interviewer. All these years later, I still have that intense determination to keep on learning and sharing that information with the world.

At this point I have seven-hundred-plus episodes of that podcast under my belt, and many of the experts I've interviewed I now consider friends. In 2012, I added a second podcast, *Ask the Low-Carb Experts,* that allows listeners to pose questions to guests specializing in a specific health topic. The curiosity of the general public about healthy living is definitely growing. It's clear that a lot of my listeners are frustrated by the often ineffective and sometimes blatantly (perhaps even deliberately) wrong or incomplete information they are receiving. They are desperate for the truth because it's their health at stake. My goal with my podcasts is to provide people with information that is accurate, up-to-date, and easy to understand, thus empowering them to become smarter patients.

Most Health Information Is Biased and Confusing

When it comes to health and medicine, the science is continually changing. If you are an informed and enlightened doctor or patient, the learning really never stops. But it can be hard to get at the truth. The pharmaceutical companies that fund research have a vested interest in certain results, so conclusions may be based on data that supports a preconceived hypothesis. And studies are often rushed, biased, or flawed—yes, sometimes even the research your doctor is basing his treatment of your health on. Furthermore, it often takes many years for the results of a study to make it to your doctor's office, so that the "latest research" your doctor is giving you may already be out of date.

Most of us get our science and health information in bits and pieces, primarily through the media. Unfortunately, one of the primary jobs of TV, radio, major newspapers, and magazines is to make money. To do that these media outlets need to generate viewers and readers by grabbing your attention; unfortunately, that often prompts them to sensationalize data and misrepresent what the research is actually saying. Therefore, it is not unusual for, say, a TV anchor or reporter to misinterpret or skew a study simply to give the story a more interesting or newsworthy angle. This makes trying to stay healthy both challenging and frustrating. How can the average Joe or Jane parse the good from the bad, the true from the false? I'm hoping this book will help when it comes to the subject of cholesterol.

Sometimes I wonder if the chaotic nature of health reporting is a deliberate tactic: Keep people utterly confused and they will simply give up trying to figure it out and just stick with the conventional wisdom we all believe is true. For example, what's the harm in taking a cholesterol-lowering medication like Lipitor or Crestor as a precaution against a heart attack? Tens of millions of other people are already opting for these "safety nets," so why not join the crowd? Here's one good reason why you shouldn't become another mindless lemming: You might not need it and it may actually be harmful to you.

Right about now some of you may be thinking, *My doctor says I have "high cholesterol" or hypercholesterolemia* (that's just a fancy term for high total and LDL cholesterol). *He says that puts me at an increased risk of developing heart disease. You don't know me, Jimmy Moore, so why should I listen to you?*

I might not know you, but I do know this: A January 2009 study published in the *American Heart Journal* found that nearly three out of four patients hospitalized for a heart attack had total cholesterol levels in the "normal" range of 200 or less. Some of them were taking statins to lower their cholesterol, and some of them had naturally low cholesterol. In other words, the statins weren't preventing heart attacks from happening, and neither was low cholesterol. As much as people would like to believe that there is some "magic pill" to address all their health concerns, especially the way statin drugs are marketed as good for your heart health, nothing like that exists. Add to that the detrimental side effects caused by "cholesterol-lowering" medications like statin drugs and you have a very troubling situation. In chapter 5, I will delve into some of the downsides of statin drugs, as well as when they should and should not be used. For now, suffice it to say that statins have some pretty serious and common side effects, including joint and muscle pain, decreased strength, and memory loss. Many people taking statins are fifty years old or older, so they might write off those symptoms as simply part of the aging process. But emerging information tells us otherwise: The very medication that is supposed to enhance and lengthen our lives may be doing just the opposite.

Drug companies won't tell you the truth about cholesterol. They are making a fortune on statins to the tune of tens of billions of dollars annually. So who will tell you the truth? And, more importantly, how can we live heart-healthy and drug-free lives?

Start by Cutting through the Misinformation

If you like straight talk that cuts through the muckity muck, you've come to the right place. The title of this book is *Cholesterol Clarity* for a reason: The intention is to make the truth about cholesterol absolutely clear. This book is not for medical geeks. It's not filled with complex terminology and jargon that makes the layperson's eyes glaze over. There are, for sure, a few technical terms you need to know, but we've provided a convenient glossary of terms in the back of the book that will explain everything for you in a language you can understand. In addition to examining the current recommendations for cholesterol levels and why they may not be valid, we will provide a practical guide to all the major cholesterol numbers, their ideal ranges (which are likely much different from what you have been told), and what specific actions in your diet and lifestyle you can take to address any troubling areas in your cholesterol profile.

The information in this book could very well be shocking and controversial, both to you *and* your doctor. The companies making money off drugs that treat high cholesterol have orchestrated a brilliant propaganda campaign. I think it's time we lifted the veil of deceit and shone a bright light on the truth.

What Makes Jimmy Moore a Cholesterol Expert?

Excellent question! Since I am merely an educated and empowered layperson with no formal training in medicine, nutrition, or any other health-related field, I expect you to question my authority to share information with you about your health. And I'm sure it doesn't help that I have just revealed that my own cholesterol levels are considered unhealthy by most medical standards. (See the 'additional resources' for my cholesterol test results from 2008 to 2013.) Additionally, I wouldn't be surprised if, based on those levels, you assume that I haven't done my homework or I don't know what I'm talking about when it comes to cholesterol. But that assumption would be wrong. In fact, I became a voracious student of this subject *because* my total cholesterol and LDL-C (the so-called "bad" cholesterol) levels have been higher than what is recommended. And in that role of student, and as a prominent health blogger and podcaster, I have had the best teachers in the world of health for nearly a decade.

It doesn't bother me at all when people question or are critical of my lack of medical and nutritional health education because I willingly admit that I don't have all the answers. But what I do have are lots of trusted advisers who know the answers to the most pressing questions about health, including my coauthor Dr. Eric Westman, MD, an internist in Durham, North Carolina who is also the co-author of the *New York Times* best-selling book *The New Atkins for a New You.* His great experience and expertise ensure that the science of cholesterol provided in this book is both insightful and up-to-date. Additionally, I tapped into my Rolodex of health experts and conducted brand-new interviews with the leading voices in the fields of health and nutrition.

I have no doubt that this book will be controversial. It challenges conventional wisdom about how we eat and live—rules that we have grown up with and followed for most of our lives. But this bears repeating: While the subject may be complicated, we have done everything possible to make it easy for you to understand. When you have finished this book, my hope is that you will know everything there is to know about cholesterol, as well as what does and does not work for real people.

Until then, hold on to your hats: We've got quite the sordid tale to unravel.

Let's Meet Your Cholesterol Experts

Through my podcasts, I have had the privilege and honor of interviewing hundreds of the best and brightest experts on a number of important health-related topics. Therefore, when I decided to write this book, I knew exactly who to call for the latest cholesterol information and advice. It gives me great pleasure to introduce these twenty-nine experts from around the world. You will find their quotes throughout the book, in sections labeled "Moment of Clarity."

Cassie Bjork, RD

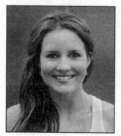

Cassie Bjork is a registered, licensed dietitian and health coach who goes by the name "Dietitian Cassie." She is passionate about helping people establish a balanced lifestyle through real, whole food and exercise. Bjork focuses on debunking diet rumors, myths, and fads, and teaches how to eat healthy by breaking down research-based material into practical forms that can be implemented by anyone. She is the cohost of the weekly iTunes health podcast *Low-Carb Conversations with Jimmy Moore & Friends*. Learn more about Bjork at:

DietitianCassie.com

Philip Blair, MD

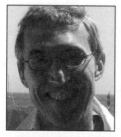

Colonel Blair (U.S. Army Retired) is a family physician providing disease management for small business employees in several states. He graduated from the U.S. Military Academy at West Point in 1972, attended the University of Miami School of Medicine, and trained as an Army family physician. After medical assignments in three continents and the Gulf War, he delivered primary care above the Arctic Circle, on Kodiak Island, and in Newfoundland. In 2002 he became vice president for disease management at Innovative Health Strategies, where he developed a highly successful interventional approach to chronic kidney disease that has saved employers over $24 million. In 2011 he formed his own company, Pro Health Advisor, providing disease management strategies that substantially improve health in over 75 percent of patients with heart or kidney disease, diabetes, obesity, and metabolic syndrome. In 2012, he met and collaborated with Dr. Duane Graveline, speaking out publically regarding the adverse effects of statin drugs and their abuse in anticholesterol therapy. Learn more about Dr. Blair at:

SpaceDoc.com/Philip_Blair_MD_Bio

Jonny Bowden, PhD

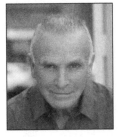 Dr. Bowden is the coauthor (with cardiologist Dr. Stephen Sinatra) of the best-selling book *The Great Cholesterol Myth: Why Lowering Cholesterol Won't Prevent Heart Disease (and the Statin-Free Plan That Will)*. Known as "The Rogue Nutritionist,"™ he was recently voted one of the hundred most influential people in health and fitness by Greatist.com. Dr. Bowden is a nationally known expert on weight loss and nutrition, a board-certified nutritionist, and the best-selling author of thirteen books on health. He is a frequent guest on television and radio, and has appeared on *The Dr. Oz Show, The Doctors,* CNN, MSNBC, Fox News, ABC, NBC, and CBS. He is a past member of the editorial advisory board of *Men's Health* magazine, nutrition editor for *Pilates Style,* and a regular contributor to *Clean Eating Magazine, Better Nutrition Magazine,* and Total Health Online. Additionally, Dr. Bowden has contributed to articles for dozens of print and online publications, including the *New York Times,* the *Wall Street Journal, Forbes, Time,* and *GQ.* He appears regularly as an expert on ABC-TV Los Angeles and serves on the scientific advisory board of several companies in the natural products industry. Learn more about Dr. Bowden at:

JonnyBowden.com

John Briffa, BSc, MB, BS

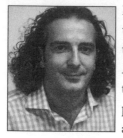

Dr. Briffa is a practicing doctor, author, and international speaker in the UK and a leading expert in nutrition and wellness. He is a former columnist for the *Daily Mail* and the *Observer,* and a regular contributor to the *Times* of London. He speaks to and facilitates programs geared to optimizing wellness, effectiveness, and sustainability for organizations in Europe and North America, and is a regular guest on radio and TV. He has authored eight books, including the best-selling *Escape the Diet Trap.* Learn more about Dr. Briffa at:

DrBriffa.com

Dominic D'Agostino, PhD

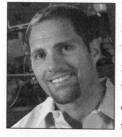

Dr. D'Agostino is an assistant professor in the Department of Molecular Pharmacology and Physiology at the University of South Florida and teaches neuropharmacology, hyperbaric medicine, medical biochemistry, and nutrition physiology. His research focuses on developing and testing ketogenic diets, calorie restriction diets, ketone esters, and ketone supplements to induce nutritional/therapeutic ketosis. These metabolic therapies can be used to treat a wide variety of disorders linked pathophysiologically to metabolic dysregulation. His research is supported by the Office of Naval Research (ONR), the Department of Defense (DoD), and private foundations working to treat and cure metabolic diseases, neurological diseases, and cancer. Learn more about Dr. D'Agostino at:

DominicDagostino.com

William Davis, MD

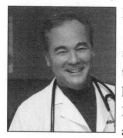

Dr. Davis is a cardiologist and author of the *New York Times* best-selling *Wheat Belly: Lose the Wheat, Lose the Weight and Find Your Path Back to Health,* the book that first exposed the dangers of genetically altered, high-yield wheat in the 1970s. He is a graduate of St. Louis University School of Medicine, with internship and residency training in internal medicine at Ohio

State University Hospitals, a fellowship in cardiovascular medicine at Ohio State University, and advanced angioplasty training at Metro Health Medical Center and Case Western Reserve University Hospitals, where he subsequently served as director of the cardiovascular fellowship and assistant professor of medicine. He presently practices cardiology in suburban Milwaukee, Wisconsin. Learn more about Dr. Davis at:

WheatBellyBlog.com

Thomas Dayspring, MD

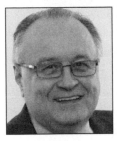

Dr. Dayspring, the director of cardiovascular education for the Foundation for Health Improvement and Technology in Richmond, Virginia, is a Fellow of both the American College of Physicians and the National Lipid Association (NLA), and is certified in lipidology and menopausal medicine by the North American Menopause Society. He is a clinical assistant professor of medicine at the University of Medicine and Dentistry of New Jersey–New Jersey Medical School. Prior to moving to Virginia, he practiced medicine in New Jersey for thirty-seven years. Dr. Dayspring has lectured far and wide on atherothrombosis, lipoprotein, and vascular biology, lipoprotein testing, and gender differences in heart disease. He has given over four thousand domestic and international lectures, including over five hundred continuing medical education (CME) programs over the last fifteen years. He is listed in the *Guide to America's Top Physicians* and is on the editorial board of the *Journal of Clinical Lipidology*. He was the recipient of the NLA's prestigious President's Award in 2011 for contributions to the field of clinical lipidology. Learn more about Dr. Dayspring at:

FHIT.org

David Diamond, PhD

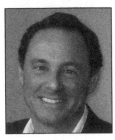

Dr. Diamond is a neuroscientist in the Departments of Psychology, Molecular Pharmacology, and Physiology at the University of South Florida, and a career scientist at the Tampa Veterans Administration Hospital. His areas of research interest include the neurobiology of learning and memory; the influence of stress on brain and behavior; animal model of post-traumatic stress disorder; the neurobiology of forgotten baby syndrome; and nutrition and health. The issue of cholesterol is personal to Dr. Diamond, who grappled with excessively high triglycerides for many years before figuring out how to achieve normal levels through nutrition. Learn more about Dr. Diamond at:

Psychology.USF.edu/faculty/diamond

Dr. Ron Ehrlich, BDS, FACNEM

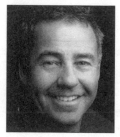

Dr. Ehrlich, one of Australia's leading holistic dentists, founded the Sydney Holistic Dental Centre (SHDC. com.au) in Sydney, Australia in 1983. He is a Fellow and board member of the Australasian College of Nutritional and Environmental Medicine (ACNEM) and is currently chairman of the organization's Advocacy and Policy Committee. Dr. Ehrlich is also cofounder and a board member of Nourishing Australia, a not-for-profit organization dedicated to informing and educating people about the critical importance of nourishing our soils, plants, animals, people, communities, and, ultimately, our planet, and inspiring them to take steps to do so. Nourishing Australia brings together holistic farm management and holistic healthcare in a soil-to-plate approach. While maintaining his clinical practice in Sydney, Dr. Ehrlich is a frequent guest speaker, regularly appears in the news media, and runs workshops for the public and health professionals on health and wellness from a unique oral health perspective. He currently cohosts a weekly podcast on iTunes called *The Good Doctors—Healthcare Unplugged*. Learn more about Dr. Ehrlich at:

DrRonEhrlich.com

Jeffry N. Gerber, MD

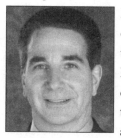

Dr. Gerber is a board-certified family physician and owner of South Suburban Family Medicine in Littleton, Colorado, where he is known as "Denver's Diet Doctor." He has been providing personalized healthcare to the local community since 1993 and continues that tradition with an emphasis on longevity, wellness, and prevention. Frustrated with spiraling healthcare costs related to the treatment of diseases like diabetes, atherosclerosis, and heart disease (just to name a few), Dr. Gerber has been focusing on prevention and treatment programs using low-carb, high-fat (LCHF), Ancestral, Paleo, and Primal diets for the overweight and obese. He maintains a database of patients and demonstrates the benefits of these types of diets by looking at their weight loss and improved cardio-metabolic markers. Redefining what healthy nutrition means is one of his primary goals. Dr. Gerber speaks frequently about these important issues to patients, the community, and other healthcare professionals. Learn more about Dr. Gerber at:

DenversDietDoctor.com

David Gillespie

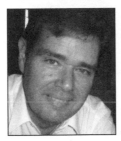

Gillespie is a Brisbane, Australia–based attorney who found that cutting out sugar from his diet reversed a lifetime of diet failure. He lost 88 pounds within eighteen months without being on a diet or exercising more: All he did was cut out sugar. Even better, the weight has stayed off for a last decade. Gillespie's experience inspired him to write *Sweet Poison*, a book that explores the science and danger of sugar addiction and consumption. He followed that up with *The Sweet Poison Quit Plan*, a step-by-step guide to cutting out sugar from your diet. In recent years, Gillespie has released *Big Fat Lies* and *Toxic Oils*; both focus on the healthy role of fat in the diet and the connection between omega-6 fats and heart disease. Learn more about Gillespie at:

SweetPoison.com.au

Duane Graveline, MD

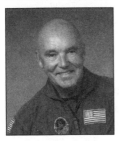

Dr. Graveline received his medical degree from the University of Vermont, interned at Walter Reed Army Hospital, and earned a master's degree in public health from Johns Hopkins University. Assigned to the Aerospace Medical Research Laboratory as a research scientist, he was designated National Aeronautics and Space Administration (NASA) flight controller for the Mercury and Gemini programs in 1962. In May 1965, he was selected as one of NASA's six scientist-astronauts. He left NASA and spent the next twenty-five years in family medical practice, taking a six-month leave in 1982 to return to NASA as chief of medical operations for the Kennedy Space Center. After retiring from medical practice, he experienced two transient global amnesia episodes after taking Lipitor, which his NASA doctors had prescribed for high cholesterol. More than a decade of research into the side effects of statins has followed. He is the author of four books on cholesterol and the side effects of statins: *Lipitor, Thief of Memory; Statin Drugs Side Effects and the Misguided War on Cholesterol; The Statin Damage Crisis;* and *The Dark Side of Statins.* Learn more about Dr. Graveline at:

SpaceDoc.com

Paul Jaminet, PhD

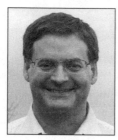

Dr. Jaminet was an astrophysicist at the Harvard-Smithsonian Center for Astrophysics before becoming a software entrepreneur during the Internet boom. He now provides strategic advice to entrepreneurial companies. Dr. Jaminet's efforts to overcome a chronic illness led him and his wife, Shou-Ching, to a seven-year research effort to refine and improve the Paleo diet, culminating in the publication of *Perfect Health Diet: Regain Health and Lose Weight by Eating the Way You Were Meant to Eat.* Since its publication, hundreds of *Perfect Health Diet* readers have cured themselves of chronic diseases, lost weight, and improved their health, mood, and overall well-being. Dr. Jaminet serves as an editor of the Ancestral Health Society's *Journal of Evolution and Health.* Learn more about Paul Jaminet at:

PerfectHealthDiet.com

Malcolm Kendrick, MD

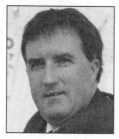

Dr. Kendrick graduated from medical school in Aberdeen, Scotland and is now a general practitioner in England. He has a special interest in the epidemiology of cardiovascular disease and has published articles in many journals, including the *British Medical Journal.* He set up the online educational system for the European Society of Cardiology, and established the first website for the National Institute for Clinical Excellence (NICE) in the UK. Dr. Kendrick has published widely on many subjects, and was elected to *Who's Who* in 2009 for his work in the area of cardiovascular medicine. He is the author of the best-selling book *The Great Cholesterol Con.* He lectures widely on a range of medical topics, and is a member of the International Network of Cholesterol Skeptics (THINCS), a group of scientists and researchers who share the belief that cholesterol does not cause cardio-vascular disease. Learn more about Dr. Kendrick at:

DrMalcolmKendrick.org

Ronald Krauss, MD

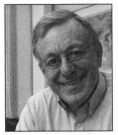

Dr. Krauss is senior scientist and director of athero-sclerosis research at Children's Hospital Oakland Research Institute, adjunct professor in the Department of Medicine at the University of California (UC) at San Francisco and in the Department of Nutritional Sciences at UC Berkeley, and guest senior scientist in the Department of Genome Sciences at Lawrence Berkeley National Laboratory. He received his undergraduate and medical degrees from Harvard University with honors. Dr. Krauss is board-certified in internal medicine, endocrinology, and metabolism, and is a member of the American Society for Clinical Investigation, a Fellow of the American Society of Nutrition and the American Heart Association (AHA), and a Distinguished Fellow of the International Atherosclerosis Society. He has served on the U.S. National Cholesterol Education Program Expert Panel on Detection, Evaluation, and Treatment of High Blood Cholesterol in Adults; was the founding chair of the AHA Council on Nutrition, Physical Activity, and Metabolism; and is a national spokesperson for the AHA. He has published over four hundred research articles and reviews on genetic, dietary, and drug effects on plasma lipoproteins and coronary artery disease. In recent years, Dr. Krauss's work has focused on the interactions of genes with dietary and drug treatments that affect metabolic phenotypes and cardiovascular disease risk. Learn more about Dr. Krauss at:

CHORI.org/Principal_Investigators/Krauss_Ronald/krauss_overview.html

Fred Kummerow, PhD

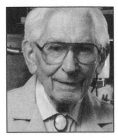

Dr. Kummerow was born on October 4, 1914, in Berlin, Germany. His family immigrated to the United States when he was nine years old, settling in Milwaukee. Dr. Kummerow attended the University of Wisconsin–Madison, where he was awarded his bachelor's in chemistry and PhD in biochemistry. From 1943 to 1945, at Clemson University in South Carolina, he worked on fortifying corn grits with niacin and iron to prevent pellagra. After resolving the pellagra crisis, he moved on to Kansas State University at Manhattan, before joining the staff of the University of Illinois at Urbana-Champaign in 1950. During his long career at the University of Illinois, he has worked tirelessly to find a cause and a cure for heart disease. Learn more about Dr. Kummerow at:

FSHN.illinois.edu

Dwight C. Lundell, MD

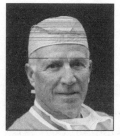

Dr. Lundell has practiced cardiovascular and thoracic surgery for over twenty-five years and was a pioneer in "off-pump" heart surgery, which reduced surgical complications and recovery times. He is in the Beating Heart Hall of Fame and has been listed in *Phoenix Magazine*'s Top Doctors issue for ten years. As a recognized leader in his field, Dr. Lundell has consulted and advised for a variety of leading medical device manufacturers. In 2005, he recognized that heart disease was largely preventable and that the focus on cholesterol was misguided. He closed his surgical practice to refocus the rest of his career on educating people about the true causes of heart disease. Dr. Lundell has written two books—*The Cure for Heart Disease* and *The Great Cholesterol Lie*—and lectures and writes about heart disease and proper human nutrition. Learn more about Dr. Lundell at:

TheCureForHeartDisease.net

Robert Lustig, MD

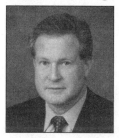

Dr. Lustig is a professor of pediatrics in the Division of Endocrinology at University of California–San Francisco (UCSF). He is a neuroendocrinologist who conducts research into and offers clinical care for patients with obesity and diabetes. Dr. Lustig graduated from MIT in 1976, and received his MD from Cornell University Medical College in 1980. He completed his pediatric residency at St. Louis Children's Hospital in 1983, and his clinical fellowship at UCSF in 1984. From there, he spent six years as a research associate in neuroendocrinology at Rockefeller University. He is the author of many academic works, and of the 2013 book *Fat Chance: Beating the*

Odds against Sugar, Processed Food, Obesity, and Disease inspired by his "Sugar: The Bitter Truth" video lecture that went viral with nearly four million views on YouTube. Dr. Lustig is also president of the nonprofit Institute for Responsible Nutrition, a think tank devoted to improving our food supply. Learn more about Dr. Lustig at:

profiles.ucsf.edu/robert.lustig

Chris Masterjohn, PhD

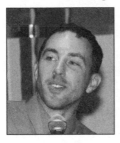

Dr. Masterjohn is the creator of a website called Cholesterol and Health, dedicated to extolling the benefits of nutrient-dense, cholesterol-rich whole foods and to elucidating the many fascinating roles that cholesterol plays in the body. He has authored several peer-reviewed publications focusing on fat-soluble vitamins, blood lipids, fatty liver disease, and heart disease. He has a PhD in nutritional sciences from the University of Connecticut and currently works as a postdoctoral research associate at the University of Illinois, where he is studying interactions between vitamins A, D, and K. His contribution to this book represents his own opinion and does not necessarily reflect the position of the University of Illinois. Learn more about Dr. Masterjohn at:

Cholesterol-And-Health.com

Donald Miller, MD

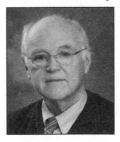

Dr. Miller is a professor of surgery and former chief of the Division of Cardiothoracic Surgery at the University of Washington School of Medicine. He received his MD degree from Harvard Medical School, did his heart surgery training at Columbia-Presbyterian Medical Center in New York, then moved to Seattle and joined the surgical faculty at the University of Washington (UW) in 1975. He currently directs the cardiothoracic surgery program at the Seattle Veterans Administration Medical Center, where he teaches UW cardiothoracic surgery residents how to perform heart surgery. Dr. Miller has researched and written articles on saturated fat, vitamin D, iodine, fluoride, and selenium, all published on LewRockwell.com. He has also written two books on heart surgery, *The Practice of Coronary Artery Bypass Surgery* and *Atlas of Cardiac Surgery*. A third, *Heart in Hand*, is

about the philosophy of Arthur Schopenhauer and his life as a heart surgeon. Learn more about Dr. Miller at:

DonaldMiller.com

Rakesh "Rocky" Patel, MD

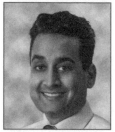

Dr. Patel is the owner of Arizona Sun Family Medicine,
PC, and is board-certified by the American Board of
Family Medicine. He received his bachelor's degree in
anthropology-zoology from the University of Michigan in 1991 and his medical degree from Wayne State
University School of Medicine in 1995. Dr. Patel completed his family medicine residency program in 1998
at Oakwood Hospital and Medical Center in Dearborn, Michigan, where
he served as the chief resident. He has been in private practice since 1998
with a primary clinical focus on the early detection and prevention of diabetes and heart disease. Learn more about Dr. Patel at:

AZPrevention.com

Fred Pescatore, MD

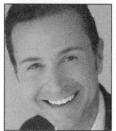

Dr. Pescatore is a traditionally trained physician who
practices nutritional medicine. He is internation-
ally recognized as a health, nutrition, and weight loss
expert. He is the author of the *New York Times* best-
selling book *The Hamptons Diet,* as well as the number-one best-selling children's health book, *Feed Your
Kids Well.* Dr. Pescatore's other books include: *Thin for
Good, The Allergy and Asthma Cure, The Hamptons Diet Cookbook,* and
Boost Your Health with Bacteria. Learn more about Dr. Pescatore at:

DrPescatore.com

Uffe Ravnskov, MD, PhD

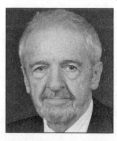

Dr. Ravnskov is an independent Danish researcher,
a member of various international scientific organizations, and a former private medical practitioner in
Sweden. In recent years he has gained notoriety for
questioning the scientific consensus regarding the lipid
hypothesis. He is a member of the free panel of the
journal of the Swedish Medical Association (the medi-

cal journal *Läkartidningen*), the International Science Oversight Board, and the International Society for the Study of Fatty Acids and Lipids, and he is the spokesman for THINCS, the International Network of Cholesterol Skeptics. He is the author of three books on the subject of cholesterol, including *The Cholesterol Myths, Ignore the Awkward: How the Cholesterol Myths are Kept Alive,* and *Fat and Cholesterol Are Good for You.* Learn more about Dr. Ravnskov at:

Ravnskov.nu/Cholesterol.htm

Stephanie Seneff, PhD

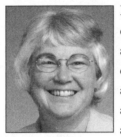

Dr. Seneff is a senior research scientist at the Massachusetts Institute of Technology's Computer Science and Artificial Intelligence Laboratory. She has a bachelor's degree from MIT in biology with a minor in food and nutrition, and a PhD in electrical engineering and computer science, also from MIT. She is the first author of several papers on theories proposing that a low-micronutrient, high-carbohydrate diet contributes to metabolic syndrome and to Alzheimer's disease, and that sulfur deficiency, environmental toxins, and insufficient exposure to sunlight play a crucial role in many modern conditions and diseases, including heart disease, diabetes, arthritis, gastrointestinal problems, and autism. She is a regular contributor to workshops hosted by the Weston A. Price Foundation, which recently honored her with the "Scientific Integrity" award. Learn more about Stephanie Seneff at:

people.csail.MIT.edu/seneff

Cate Shanahan, MD

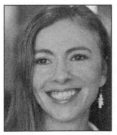

Dr. Shanahan is a family physician and national authority on longevity and nutrition. Trained in biochemistry and genetics at Cornell, she has two decades of experience examining the effects of industrial ingredients on individuals and across generations as they interfere with metabolism, genetic expression, joint function, brain health, and skeletal development. She is the author of two books: *Deep Nutrition: Why Your Genes Need Traditional Food* and *Food Rules: A Doctor's Guide to Healthy Eating.* She designed the

Los Angeles Lakers' new diet, and, for the benefit of adults and children everywhere, is working to make well-sourced foods cooler than sugary sports drinks. Learn more about Dr. Shanahan at:

DrCate.com

Ken Sikaris, BSc, MBBS, FRCPA, FAACB, FFSc

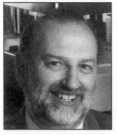

Dr. Sikaris is a science and medicine graduate of Melbourne University in Australia. He also trained as a medical specialist in chemical pathology before taking his first position as director of chemical pathology at St Vincent's Hospital in Melbourne, which included supervising a specialized lipid (cholesterol) laboratory. He has also been involved in lipid research and practiced in a lipid clinic. For the last twenty years he has worked in private pathology companies and supervises the blood testing of thousands of patients every day. He currently works with Sonic Healthcare, the third largest pathology company in the world, where he is clinical support services director. He is also an associate professor in the Department of Pathology at Melbourne University. Learn more about Dr. Sikaris at:

MPS.com.au/about-us/pathologists/pr-list/dr-ken-sikaris.aspx

Patty Siri-Tarino, PhD

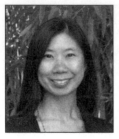

Dr. Siri-Tarino is associate staff scientist and program director of the Family Heart and Nutrition Center at Children's Hospital Oakland & Research Center Oakland. She is interested in bringing nutritional research to the community and empowering people through education and skills training, including mindfulness and meditation, to live happily and well. Her research expertise is in the mechanisms underlying the dyslipidemia associated with insulin resistance and obesity. Dr. Siri-Tarino has designed and conducted clinical trials evaluating dietary and pharmacological modulators of lipid profiles. Most recently, she coauthored several publications reevaluating the association of saturated fat with cardiovascular disease risk. Dr. Siri-Tarino holds a BS in biology and German area studies from Tufts University, an MS in epidemiology from Erasmus University in the Netherlands, and a PhD in nutrition from Columbia University. Learn more about Dr. Siri-Tarino at:

CHORI.org

Mark Sisson

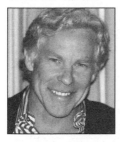

Mark Sisson is a leading authority in the low-carb movement, as well as an expert in evolution-based health, fitness, and nutrition. A noted researcher, author, and lecturer, he has dedicated his personal and professional life to offering sustainable solutions for health, wellness, and weight loss. He is the author of the Amazon best-seller *The Primal Blueprint*. He is also the founder and CEO of Primal Nutrition, Inc., a provider of health education materials and lifestyle-enhancing nutritional supplements. Sisson attended Williams College, where he received a BA degree with a major in biology. As an elite endurance athlete, he finished fifth in the 1980 USA National Marathon Championships (2:18:01) and fourth in the 1982 Hawaii Ironman Triathlon. Learn more about Mark Sisson at:

MarksDailyApple.com

Gary Taubes

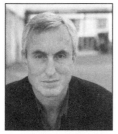

Gary Taubes is a contributing correspondent for *Science* magazine. His writing has appeared in *The Atlantic*, *The New York Times Magazine*, *Esquire*, and *The Best of the Best American Science Writing* (2010). He has received three Science in Society Journalism Awards from the National Association of Science Writers, the only print journalist so recognized. Gary is currently a Robert Wood Johnson Foundation Investigator in Health Policy Research at the University of California, Berkeley School of Public Health. He is the author of the *New York Times* bestselling books *Good Calories Bad Calories* and *Why We Get Fat And What To Do About It* exposing the story about how we have been misled about diet, weight loss and health. Gary is also the co-founder of the Nutrition Science Initiative (NuSi), a non-profit 501(c)(3) whose purpose is to facilitate and fund rigorous, well-controlled experiments targeted at resolving unambiguously many of the outstanding nutrition controversies—to answer the question definitively of what constitutes a healthy diet. Learn more about Gary Taubes at:

GaryTaubes.com

These are my cream-of-the-crop experts on the subject of cholesterol. Additionally, my coauthor, Eric Westman, MD, will be sharing his thoughts in the "Doctor's Note" entries scattered throughout the book. Here's his first!

DOCTOR'S NOTE FROM DR. ERIC WESTMAN: It's a pleasure for me to coauthor this book with Jimmy Moore as we help you make sense of your blood cholesterol numbers. I've known Jimmy for many years now and witnessed his own amazing journey. I can personally attest to his grasp of this subject.

Don't worry if some of the "Moment of Clarity" quotes from my expert friends are too complex for you to fully understand. I will explain all the relevant basic information you need to know in a language you can grasp, embrace, and employ in your own life, and there's also a convenient glossary of terms at the back of this book to help you along the way if you're curious to learn more. So how about we jump right in? Cholesterol clarity begins right here, right now!

Chapter 1

What Is Cholesterol and Why Do You Need It?

For decades, well-meaning health professionals have told us that we don't need cholesterol or that having a lot of it is bad. Drug therapies have been developed specifically to combat this problem. It might therefore strike you as funny that in this chapter I'm going to tell you why you *do* need it. But here's the simple truth: Your body could not survive without cholesterol.

MOMENT OF CLARITY: "Cholesterol is essential for our bodies to function and without cholesterol you would die. In fact, the majority of the cholesterol in our blood comes from our own bodies making it. I don't think a lot of people understand that concept. People mistakenly think they get most of their cholesterol from their food and that's not true. Cholesterol is used to make hormones like estrogen and testosterone, is transported into the adrenal gland to aid in hormone synthesis, repair nerves, and make bile for fat digestion, it's a structural component of our cells, it synthesizes vitamin D—it plays such a critical role in our body that we genuinely need it. If our levels of cholesterol are too low, that can play a negative role in our health, too, as a telltale sign of autoimmune disease or even cancer."

-Cassie Bjork

MOMENT OF CLARITY: "Cholesterol is one of the most important molecules in the human body: we would die very quickly without it. It's involved in the creation of vitamin D and in the formation of many important sex hormones, it's an integral part of cell membranes, and it's necessary for the production of bile, which is critical to our ability to emulsify and digest fats."

– Mark Sisson

Cholesterol is a waxy, fatlike substance produced primarily in the liver. It is absolutely essential to the life of humans and animals; without it, our cells could not repair themselves, we could not maintain proper hormone levels, we could not properly absorb vitamin D from the sun, we could not regulate our salt and water balance, and we could not digest fats. And, oh yes, it also improves memory and boosts levels of serotonin—the chemical that makes us happy. Cholesterol sounds like it's pretty important, don't you think? But wait, there's more.

MOMENT OF CLARITY: "Chemically, the cholesterol in your blood and the cholesterol in the foods you eat are the same thing, since there is only one molecule that would be identified as cholesterol. But that doesn't mean that most of the cholesterol inside your body is coming from your food. The reason for this is that we have a certain need for cholesterol and we regulate that need for cholesterol fairly tightly. So if we eat a lot of cholesterol, our bodies make less of it; if we eat less cholesterol, our bodies make more of it. In most people, the majority of cholesterol that is circulating in their blood is made by their own bodies. The amount of cholesterol-containing foods they eat isn't going to have a big impact on their blood cholesterol levels. It can vary from person to person, but in general the cholesterol in your diet is never the major determinant of cholesterol levels in the blood or in the body."

— Dr. Chris Masterjohn

In April 2013, I attended a medical conference of the American Society of Bariatric Physicians in San Diego. One of the speakers, Peter Attia, MD, gave a talk called "The Straight Dope on Cholesterol" (google that phrase to read his ten-part blog series on the subject), and he made a fascinating point: Only 15 percent of the cholesterol that you consume through diet is absorbed and used by the body; the other 85 percent is excreted. His natural conclusion? The cholesterol we consume has very little to do with the cholesterol levels in our bloodstream. That salient point really stuck with me in light of all the hysteria about eliminating cholesterol-rich foods from our diet.

Did you know that cholesterol has some amazing antioxidant properties that can actually help guard you against heart disease? Ironic, isn't it? There are many reasons why your cholesterol levels might go up: It could be your body's response to inflammation (a critical concept we'll discuss in chapter 2), or it could be a sign that part of your body is malfunctioning—maybe, for example, your thyroid function is low. We'll get into these and the other possible reasons for elevated cholesterol levels later on in the book. For now, all you need to know is that cholesterol is a major line of defense when your immune system comes under attack. So lowering cholesterol levels artificially with drugs could make you more susceptible to germs or bacteria wreaking havoc on your health. Are you getting more excited about cholesterol? Maybe just a little?

MOMENT OF CLARITY: "LDL [low-density lipoprotein] particles serve as your body's scouts or sentinels, detecting foreign threats like germs. The LDL particle protein is very fragile and very easily oxidized. When it comes in contact with bacterial cell wall components, it quickly becomes oxidized LDL, which doesn't get taken up by cells that are looking to take in fats. Instead, oxidized LDL gets taken up by the white blood cells, and an appropriate immune response is mounted against the microbe that oxidized the LDL lipoprotein. That's why high levels of oxidized LDL are associated with a lot of health problems. It means you have a lot of foreign things that shouldn't be inside you stimulating your immune system."

– Paul Jaminet

But I'm Still Worried about Cholesterol "Clogging" My Arteries

MOMENT OF CLARITY: "I think the cholesterol theory is actually quite persuasive at face value. If you tease away what's inside a clogged artery, you find cholesterol, and this can make the role of cholesterol in heart disease appear like an open-and-shut case. Obviously atherosclerotic plaque is much more complex than just cholesterol. But the very fact that it's there, along with evidence in certain populations linking high cholesterol with heart disease, helps to make the cholesterol hypothesis very plausible, I think, at least at first sight."

– Dr. John Briffa

It seems to make logical sense: Eat a lot of saturated fat and cholesterol and it will clog your arteries, much like greasy sludge clogs the pipes in a kitchen sink. It's a convenient and vivid image. But it's also dead wrong because your arteries are nothing like the pipes under your sink. The last time I checked, normal body temperature was approximately 98.6 degrees Fahrenheit, and that would melt saturated fat. It would be the same as putting a block of butter on your front porch on a hot day. Before long, you'd find a big puddle of melted butter.

MOMENT OF CLARITY: "The way the body transports fats and cholesterol into the body is really interesting because it doesn't go directly into the bloodstream from the gut. Instead, it gets shipped through the lymph nodes and it arrives right at the big vein that goes into the heart. Basically, it wants to direct cholesterol and fat toward the heart to give it first dibs. The body has to make sure the heart gets plenty of this first because it knows the heart needs fat and cholesterol. The heart is eager to get dietary cholesterol and fat, and the gut stands ready to give it to the heart. That's got to be by design to tell us that the heart needs cholesterol and fat. Everything else just goes straight to the liver before being used elsewhere in the body."

— Stephanie Seneff

Dr. Michael Rothberg of the Cleveland Clinic is the author of "Coronary Artery Disease as Clogged Pipes: A Misconceptual Model," an article that appeared in the January 2013 issue of the American Heart Association's scientific journal *Circulation: Cardiovascular Qualities and Outcomes*. He wrote it in response to a provocative health advertisement he had seen in the *New York Times Magazine*, which had used the clogged-pipe imagery as a way to promote a cardiac catheterization lab. Yes, the imagery is "simple, familiar, and evocative," he noted in the article. Unfortunately, he added, "it is also wrong."

Ancel Keys and the Lipid Hypothesis: A Brief History of Misinformation

MOMENT OF CLARITY: "Nobody cared very much about cholesterol until the Korean War when we saw a very high percentage of young people with significant atherosclerotic plaque. Everybody then got excited and started looking into this. We had known for long time that this plaque contained cholesterol, along with other cellular debris. This is when the focus turned to cholesterol."

— Dr. Dwight Lundell

MOMENT OF CLARITY: "We have this issue of cholesterol being the number-one cause of heart disease in the eyes of most of my cardiologist colleagues. That would have some merit if it was 1963."

— Dr. William Davis

In 1856, the German pathologist Rudolf Virchow first proposed that the accumulation of cholesterol inside the arterial walls of human beings leads to the development of atherosclerosis and heart disease. The idea gained a little traction in 1913, when a Russian pathologist named Nikolai Anitschkow found that feeding cholesterol to rabbits led to the development of atherosclerotic plaque. (The fact that rabbits mostly consume a vegetarian diet and therefore are not biologically adapted to eating foods with cholesterol was never brought up.) But the publication of George Duff and Gardner McMillian's article "Lipid Hypothesis," published in the *American Journal of Medicine* in 1951, really got the anticholesterol ball rolling.

The Lipid Hypothesis captured the attention of an American scientist named Ancel Keys, who is widely considered the "father" of the cholesterol-heart hypothesis. In 1956, the American Heart Association endorsed Keys's Seven Countries Study, which purported to prove that cardiovascular disease is caused by the consumption of dietary fat and cholesterol (Keys, by the way, went on to popularize the Mediterranean diet that is still promoted as healthy today). I'll be delving more deeply into the intricate and unfortunate role Keys played in the cholesterol story later, but you can find plenty more about his flawed science in Tom Naughton's hilarious and informative documentary film *Fat Head*, and in the book *Good Calories, Bad Calories*, by *New York Times* best-selling science writer Gary Taubes (one of this book's experts). Both of these detail how Keys fudged his data to fit his own hypothesis.

The vilification of dietary fat reached a fever pitch with the Coronary Primary Prevention Trial (CPPT), which was backed by the National Institutes of Health, and ran from 1973 through 1984. Based on this trial's results, a low-fat, low-cholesterol diet—combined with cholesterol-lowering medications—was recommended for heart health. But, again, the study was flawed; the behind-the-scenes shenanigans involved were utterly unscrupulous. However, the brainwashing had already begun; Americans were advised to cut their fat intake significantly—by doctors, government agencies, manufacturers of food, and the media. Anyone who cared about their health in the decades that followed obediently followed this completely unproven advice.

Based on the CPPTs faulty data, the NIH boldly stated that no more trials were necessary: "We have proved that it is worthwhile to lower blood cholesterol ... Now is the time for treatment." The American Heart Association echoed that sentiment in a separate statement. Together they encouraged pharmaceutical companies to begin developing what would later become statin drugs. Calling this the single biggest blunder in the history of medicine is not overstating the case. And we're still reaping what we have sown three decades later.

Failing to challenge the belief popularized by Keys and the CPPT—that eating saturated fat will raise your cholesterol and clog your arteries—has led to several unintended consequences, key among them that the diets of Americans have changed, mostly for the worse. Statistics from the U.S. Department of Agriculture's Economic Research Service between 1977 and 1978 and 2005 and 2008 show that Americans dutifully cut their fat intake from 85.6 g to 75.2 g daily. Additionally, over the same periods, the percentage of total calories consumed from fat fell from 39.7 percent to 33.4 percent. And what has happened to the rates of obesity, diabetes, and heart disease since then? You already know the answer: Heart disease is now the number-one killer of both men and women, and nearly one million Americans have heart attacks annually. Obesity and diabetes have reached epidemic proportions. The financial burden of coronary artery disease alone totals close to $110 billion a year, and that trend is growing.

If dietary fat and cholesterol consumption are the true culprits in heart disease as we've been led to believe, then how can this be happening? The answer is obvious: They are *not* the true culprits. Emerging evidence proves that these supposed health experts have been dead wrong and yet they continue to cling to this outdated and outright harmful information. You may have noticed that experts don't like to be challenged or admit they are wrong; they generally need to see overwhelming evidence to the contrary to change their opinions. The good news is that, in the case of cholesterol, the evidence is mounting, slowly but surely. It's only a matter of time.

MOMENT OF CLARITY: "Dietary cholesterol is not the problem. We've shown that in a study I published in the January 1979 issue of the *American Journal of Clinical Nutrition*. What we showed in that research is that you don't induce heart disease by consuming dietary cholesterol."

— Dr. Fred Kummerow

Your Number-One Health Advocate Is YOU

MOMENT OF CLARITY: "The population will become split between the smart and the dumb. The smart ones will begin taking their health into their own hands because they're already seeing that what we are doing now is not working. Our diet is not working because 70 percent of us are overweight and obese, we have 29 million diabetics and 75 million more prediabetics, and the rest of us don't even know we're prediabetic! People are realizing that what we are doing is not working and they are looking for other ways around this. That's where do-it-yourself healthcare and self-monitoring will become the norm."

— Dr. Dwight Lundell

I am a huge proponent of people taking responsibility for their own health. We are all unique individuals with different needs and yet we are treated like lemmings by the medical profession when it comes to our health. I get why so many people abdicate personal responsibility with their health; it's so much easier to just do what we're told. But that approach clearly doesn't work: Science changes all the time, and medical and nutrition specialists simply can't keep up. How can they possibly have all the answers? Food and drug companies don't care about your health; they are quite simply motivated by profit under the illusion they are making you healthier. Unfortunately, they are not. There's no way around it: If you want to be healthy, it's up to you to make it happen! Educate yourself, and then act on what you learn. You must be the final arbiter of your own health.

MOMENT OF CLARITY: "Most doctors are horrified when they meet a patient who is eating a low-carb, high-fat diet. They usually tell him that there is a great risk that very soon he will die from heart disease. But a patient who has slimmed down, whose laboratory values have become normal, and who has been able to skip his insulin and diabetes drugs by following this diet, should not listen to such warnings."

— Dr. Uffe Ravnskov

MOMENT OF CLARITY: "I can remember back in the 1960s, there wasn't any problem eating lard or having lots of fat on your meat. And sweets were like a treat. You only had dessert or even a soft drink at parties and on special occasions."

— Dr. Ken Sikaris

Cholesterol and blood test terminology are explained later in the book. But for now the one word you need to know about is *inflammation*, which we will address in the next chapter. This is the real culprit in heart disease, not cholesterol. Without inflammation in the body, cholesterol would move freely through the body and never accumulate on the walls of blood vessels. Inflammation is caused when we expose our bodies to toxins or foods the human body wasn't designed to process. These foods, however, are not the saturated fats in butter and meat and cheese—the things we've been taught to avoid. They are foods marketed as "heart-healthy." How scary is that? Blaming cholesterol for heart disease is like saying that firefighters cause fires! Being at the scene of the accident doesn't make you culpable.

MOMENT OF CLARITY: "The idea of the continued promotion of LDL cholesterol as the culprit in heart disease is to keep it simple and stick with what the physicians already know. The thinking is that there's no sense in complicating things or making the tests any more expensive than they already are. This is about the maximal bang for the buck, and the authorities in this field tend to toy believe that sticking with LDL cholesterol gives them that, and that they are doing the best job for the patients. If you misdiagnose a few patients here and there, that's the price you have to pay in life."

— Gary Taubes

KEY CHOLESTEROL CLARITY CONCEPTS

→ **Your body *needs* cholesterol to survive.**

→ **Cholesterol plays many important roles in the health of your body.**

→ **The "clogged arteries" concept is dead wrong.**

→ **People have dutifully cut their fat intake, but heart disease rates have grown.**

→ **You are your own best health advocate.**

Chapter 2
Forget Cholesterol— It's the Inflammation

MOMENT OF CLARITY: "The idea of cholesterol being dangerous has become such a deep part of our culture that it is now automatically synonymous with cardio-metabolic risk. Until we make a change in our thinking about cholesterol, it will be difficult to convince people. And frankly, you've got to first convince a lot of medical providers to shift those particular terms because we can't seem to get away from the idea that cholesterol is the bad guy. As long as we continue to use derogatory terms about cholesterol, the confusion will go on."

– Dr. Philip Blair

MOMENT OF CLARITY: "We've long known that atherosclerosis is an inflammatory disease. In the absence of inflammation or injury to the endothelial cell, the cholesterol would never go through the arterial wall and it would never stay there."

– Dr. Dwight Lundell

In the first chapter I stated that there is a lack of evidence supporting commonly held beliefs about cholesterol's role in heart disease. Many of you are probably still skeptical, and you should be. One of the purposes of this book is to encourage you to challenge everything you read and hear from experts so that you can become an active participant in your own healthcare.

But people like Dr. Westman and I are not alone in challenging commonly held beliefs. There is a growing group of empowered patients, as well as members of the medical and health community (like the many experts quoted in this book), who are rejecting the scientific premise of the cholesterol-heart hypothesis. And, incidentally, note the word *hypothesis*: This theory about cholesterol has never been proven!

MOMENT "If you had asked me twenty years ago if I thought blood cholesterol **OF CLARITY:** levels were critically important, I would have said yes. But now my views have changed. What's the difference? Not that I was a bad person then and I'm a better person now. I just wasn't very up on the science then and I believe I'm more up on it now. I was misguided, but I wasn't intentionally trying to mislead anyone. Unfortunately, I believe there are a lot of medical professionals who are in this category."

– Dr. John Briffa

It's no mystery why you and millions of others are still concerned about elevated cholesterol levels. And you *should* know what your cholesterol test results mean, including which markers are most important to pay attention to and how you can optimize your health by improving those numbers. I'll get into that later. But first, let's take a closer look at inflammation—the root cause of the rise in heart attacks, strokes, and cardiovascular disease.

Without Inflammation, Cholesterol Can't Harm You

MOMENT "When we're talking about inflammation, I like to look at what's **OF CLARITY:** causing it. If the client's C-reactive protein levels are high, I want to look for the root cause of the inflammation and what's causing the damage. Things like smoking, excessive alcohol consumption, consuming trans fats and processed carbohydrates, having high blood sugar levels, chemical exposure, high blood pressure, and stress can all contribute to this. Everything on this list is very different than blaming inflammation on a high-fat diet, which is what many trusted professionals will point their finger at right away."

– Cassie Bjork

When most people hear the word *inflammation*, they think about the time they twisted their ankle or broke their arm and the area became swollen, with heat and pain radiating from the source of the injury. This temporary condition, known as acute inflammation, is a quick, direct response to injuries and is designed to speed up the process of healing. Chronic inflammation, by contrast, is slower and far more damaging; it happens over many years and is caused by, among other things, poor diet, smoking, lack of sleep, infrequent exercise, elevated stress, and compromised gut health. This is the inflammation that brings on heart disease.

Let's be clear: Inflammation is a good thing; it is an excellent natural defense against bacteria, viruses, fungi, and toxins. It only becomes dangerous and life-threatening when it is chronically elevated over long periods. The importance of chronic inflammation was highlighted in Dr. Dwight Lundell's outstanding article "Heart Surgeon Speaks Out on What Really Causes Heart Disease," which was published on the website *Sign of The Times* in March 2012. In the article, Dr. Lundell noted that, in the absence of inflammation, "Cholesterol would move freely throughout the body as nature intended." Unfortunately, chronic inflammation has become the norm for most people living in America and in westernized cultures around the world.

DOCTOR'S NOTE FROM DR. ERIC WESTMAN: When I was in
    medical school, one of my professors would say, "Half of what
    we are teaching you now will be proven to be wrong. The
    problem is that we don't know which half it is." It is time
    to add 'cholesterol is bad' to the half that was proven to be
    wrong.

One of the blood markers that we'll be examining later in the book is high-sensitivity C-reactive protein (hs-CRP). This is the primary inflammation marker for determining the amount of chronic inflammation in your body—the cause of heart disease and other health complications—and therefore much more important than your low-density lipoprotein (LDL) and total cholesterol levels, the markers most commonly tested. Any physician or medical lab can test your levels of hs-CRP, and yet I'm going to guess that you've probably never even heard of it.

Despite all the emerging evidence that inflammation is the key marker for heart disease, and that identifying and treating it with changes in nutrition, exercise, and lifestyle are the critical first steps in battling heart disease, major health groups continue to blame cholesterol. Their misguided advice is discussed in the next chapter.

KEY CHOLESTEROL CLARITY CONCEPTS

→ Be skeptical about what you have been told about cholesterol.

→ Chronic inflammation from elevated CRP levels is the major cause of heart disease.

→ Cholesterol cannot accumulate in your arteries without inflammation.

→ Levels of high-sensitivity C-reactive protein is the key marker for chronic inflammation, and yet it is rarely tested.

Chapter 3

What Do Major Health Groups Say about Cholesterol?

MOMENT OF CLARITY: "The whole system has gone berserk. They've created this incredibly misleading house of cards of nutritional information and how heart disease is caused. They have constructed this rickety structure that is supposed to support the treatment of heart disease. The problem is that there is a germ of truth to all of this, so it's not like the whole idea was concocted out of the blue to purposely mislead people. But there are so many problems with the entire message. It's hard to take the four numbers on a typical lipid panel and try to squeeze any real, meaningful truth out of it."

— Dr. William Davis

DOCTOR'S NOTE FROM DR. ERIC WESTMAN: Experts have naively assumed that cholesterol and fat buildup on the arteries is reduced by lowering the cholesterol and fat in the diet. This logic is like watching the sun go across the sky and assuming that the sun goes around the earth. "We" believed that for a long, long time, before the ingenuity and telescopes of the astronomers found out otherwise!

The major health organizations have reasons for both their misguided assumptions about cholesterol and the promotion of them, which we'll get into later. Before we do, let's take a look at the positions of America's most prominent health groups, and the conventional wisdom they promote regarding diet, cholesterol, and heart disease risks.

United States Department
of Health and Human Services (HHS)

The HHS is the government agency ostensibly in charge of vetting all the science related to health. Through this process, HHS officials determine the best course of action for optimal health. They have something called the National Cholesterol Education Program that seeks to teach us about cholesterol and the role it plays in our health. Unfortunately, what they are teaching has very little to do with improving health.

The HHS contends that blood cholesterol "has a lot to do with your chances of getting heart disease" and that having elevated levels of cholesterol in your blood is "one of the major risk factors for heart disease." They add that, "the higher your blood cholesterol level, the greater your risk for developing heart disease or having a heart attack." These definitive statements are based on their belief that when cholesterol builds up in the walls of your arteries, the process of "hardening" (atherosclerosis) begins. The arteries slowly become too narrow for blood to flow to the heart, and finally become blocked, which can result in a heart attack or heart failure. This is why the HHS urges Americans to lower their high cholesterol by any means necessary.

MOMENT OF CLARITY: "We are constantly being bombarded by messages that encourage and maintain this cultural myth about cholesterol being linked to heart disease. It's a myth that has been perpetuated for the past fifty years, and it keeps being reinforced time and time again."

– Dr. Philip Blair

United States Centers for Disease Control (CDC)

Go to the CDC website and click on "Heart Disease Conditions," which includes this position on heart disease: When there is "too much" cholesterol in the blood coming from saturated fat and cholesterol in your diet, LDL cholesterol begins to deposit in your arteries, leading to constricted blood flow to the heart. This, the CDC warns, can lead to a heart attack, stroke, even death. So CDC officials, too, blame the saturated fat and cholesterol in the food you consume for putting you at risk, and they advise people to eat less fat and cholesterol, thus lowering LDL and preventing the possibility of heart disease.

MOMENT OF CLARITY: "There's a lot of brainwashing going on in health. Just as all calories are not the same, all fats are not the same and all cholesterol particles are not the same. But people don't get it because they are easily swayed. I'm a scientist and I get it. My job is to bring the science to the people. Some get it, but most don't. That makes them easy prey for the marketers."

– Dr. Robert Lustig

MOMENT OF CLARITY: "The conventional wisdom on heart disease is too simplistic and dated. The public health authorities, the American Heart Association and other groups, locked themselves in when they started giving dietary advice in the 1970s and 1980s, and that's the last thing you want to do in science. The root of all episodes of bad science stems from turning assumptions into facts and endorsing them prematurely. And if you then act on these assumptions, as happens in medicine and public health, you lock yourself in further, without ever finding out if what you're doing is actually the right thing. "

– Gary Taubes

American Heart Association (AHA)

You would think that a group like the AHA would stay on top of all the latest and best information related to heart health. After all, the association's little heart symbol is plastered across all kinds of food products in grocery stores; a subtle yet tacit endorsement that what you are about to eat is healthy. While AHA officials do acknowledge that cholesterol is beneficial to the human body, they simultaneously claim that foods with saturated and trans fat can increase your blood cholesterol levels too much, leading to cardiovascular disease. They therefore advise you to limit your consumption of those foods, including cholesterol-heavy egg yolks. Do you know how many essential nutrients are in an egg yolk? A lot. But it's better to just cut them out of your diet than risk raising your cholesterol, right?

MOMENT OF CLARITY: "The yolk of an egg is incredibly nutritious. It contains 100 percent of the carotenoids; essential fatty acids; fat-soluble vitamins A, E, D, and K that our body requires; and more than 90 percent of the calcium, iron, phosphorus, zinc, thiamine, folate, B12, pantothenic acid, as well as the majority of the copper, manganese, and selenium our body requires. They are also excellent sources of lutein and zeaxanthin, which evidence has shown are highly protective against developing macular degeneration—the major cause of blindness in the elderly. Since most people don't eat liver, egg yolks are the only major source of choline, which helps to protect against fatty liver disease, which afflicts about one-third of Americans. Additionally, animal studies indicate that when you get three times more than the recommended amount of choline early in life, you can have lifelong protection against senility and dementia, along with major boosts in memory and mental performance throughout your life. Eggs yolks are primarily feared by people because of their cholesterol content, but they are jam-packed with really important nutrients, some of which are very difficult to get anywhere else in your diet."

— Dr. Chris Masterjohn

DOCTOR'S NOTE FROM DR. ERIC WESTMAN: I think eggs just might be the perfect food. Think about it: An egg is a whole baby chicken, which makes it a complete nutritional package.

American Medical Association (AMA)

This prominent physicians' group promotes its "Healthier Life Steps" program for patients and its "healthy eating" guidelines—the same ones promoted by the U.S. Department of Agriculture (USDA) and the USDA's MyPlate nutritional advice. These include some smart advice for overall health: Don't smoke, eat a lot of vegetables, exercise, and limit consumption of alcohol. But for heart health the AMA falls back on the popular and misguided panacea of a low-fat, high-carb diet.

MOMENT OF CLARITY: "We start with this mess of telling people to cut the fat, cut the saturated fat, and then follow with cholesterol panels. But cutting fat does not reduce the risk of heart disease. In fact, eating a low-fat diet causes incredible metabolic distortions, like high blood sugar, hyperglycemia, rising fasting glucose, insulin resistance, growth of belly fat, hypertension, metabolic syndrome, and diabetes in the genetically susceptible."

— Dr. William Davis

The Mayo Clinic

The Mayo Clinic states very clearly on its website that healthy arterial health depends on your arteries remaining flexible and elastic. This is an accurate statement. They go on to explain that pressure in the arteries can make the walls thick and stiff, which results in restrictive blood flow to vital organs like your heart. Again, this is perfectly fine. However, when the Mayo Clinic doctors state that "hardening of the arteries," or atherosclerosis, is brought on by the "buildup of fats and cholesterol in and on your artery walls," they are perpetuating the fallacy of conventional wisdom regarding dietary fat and cholesterol. Are you sensing a theme yet?

MOMENT OF CLARITY: "What we're fighting against is the idea that dietary fat clogging arteries is the problem. Even lipid scientists who understand that inflammation is a problem are still talking about particle numbers as if there is something inherent in fat that makes it clog our arteries. And that is not correct. What happens is we lose the function of the lipoproteins to deliver fats to cells and tissues. So fat doesn't clog our arteries like what happens in the pipes underneath your sink. This kind of thinking is absurd, given the fact that we now know that fat does not travel in these little blobs of fat in our arteries. It's completely encased in lipoproteins, which are fat-soluble. It cannot clog our arteries any more than red blood cells can clog our arteries."

— Dr. Cate Shanahan

The Cleveland Clinic

This prestigious research facility claims that elevated levels of low-density lipoprotein (LDL) are "a major cause of heart disease." In the opinion of the Cleveland Clinic researchers, LDL leads to a "buildup of fatty deposits within your arteries, reducing or blocking the flow of blood and oxygen your heart needs." According to their website, when this happens you feel chest pain and may experience a heart attack. Their primary advice for preventing heart disease: Lower LDL by any means necessary, including the aggressive use of pharmaceutical drug therapies, such as statins.

The Cleveland Clinic adds that it is "extremely important for everyone—men and women of every age, with or without known heart disease—to have a low LDL level," which they define as below 100 mg/dL. For "better outcomes," they recommend lowering it to 60 mg/dL. Interestingly, they also encourage lower levels of C-reactive protein, the key inflammation marker we discussed in the previous chapter. They do not, however, point out that one is more important than the other.

MOMENT OF CLARITY: "It seemed like however you altered the LDL particle, it became atherogenic. And this still seemed to support the whole cholesterol hypothesis because all these forms of LDL were cholesterol-rich particles. So when the statin drugs were coming into play in the early 1990s, it was thought to be consistent that if you just stop making those LDL particles—no matter what changes them—then you'll decrease the risk of disease."

– Dr. Ken Sikaris

As you can see, all these highly regarded organizations—each considered a major authority on health—have formed a united front when it comes to the cause of heart disease. And the message they are promulgating goes like this: Including saturated fat and cholesterol in your diet leads to an increase in LDL, thus putting you at a greater risk of heart attack or stroke. To avoid this, bring your cholesterol levels down by reducing consumption of saturated fat and cholesterol, and when that's not enough, take a prescription medication to make it happen.

How convenient that so many doctors, dietitians, and know-it-all gurus believe the exact same thing. Too bad that it is all predicated on misguided reasoning, though. In the next chapter, we'll learn more about the countermovement to the cholesterol hypothesis that is growing in the medical community.

MOMENT OF CLARITY: "Cholesterol has been wrongly vilified for an alleged association with an increased risk for heart disease. Over the years we have learned that this association is loose at best and nonexistent at worst. Nevertheless, people tend to believe what they've read for years or have been told by their doctors, despite new evidence. A few erroneous assumptions, followed by bits of skewed data, followed by a public policy machine eager to find a villain in a scary epidemic of heart disease—that's the genesis of the cholesterol-heart hypothesis we're still stuck with. And at some point it became difficult to speak out in favor of cholesterol as a possible good guy."

– Mark Sisson

DOCTOR'S NOTE FROM DR. ERIC WESTMAN: I'm optimistic that one day we will teach that fat in the diet is a good thing because our bodies need fat for vital functions and for making us feel full. We made this point in *The New Atkins for a New You*, with a chapter called "Fat is Your Friend."

KEY CHOLESTEROL CLARITY CONCEPTS

→ **Health authorities have formed a united front in support of the cholesterol-heart hypothesis.**

→ **They would have you believe that eating saturated fat is harmful because it raises cholesterol.**

Chapter 4

Doctors Are Questioning the Anticholesterol Message

MOMENT OF CLARITY: "Over the past decade we have found that cholesterol causality is nothing but a massive con job organized by Big Pharma. Cholesterol has nothing to do with atherosclerosis, which helps to explain why, in over half of new heart attacks, the cholesterol levels are normal or well below normal."

— Dr. Duane Graveline

Good news! Yes, there is a lot of resistance to change in the medical and nutrition communities. But there are also a growing number of enlightened doctors and dietitians who are questioning the reliability and accuracy of the anticholesterol message. They have observed the failure of cholesterol-lowering strategies either in their patients and clients or, in some cases, in their own bodies. Could all the time and energy invested in the idea that cholesterol is linked to heart disease have been a complete waste of time? Some are beginning to think so.

MOMENT OF CLARITY: "The cholesterol myths continue because of the money involved. The statin industry is such a big, big moneymaker that they don't want to burst that bubble. I think there must be plenty of people in those industries who know that statins are bad but they're keeping it under wraps. I cannot believe that they wouldn't know because it just seems so obvious to me. The cholesterol story is a very easy story for people to understand. It's dead wrong, but it's easy for people to understand and believe that high cholesterol clogs the arteries and causes the heart to have problems. This is how statins have been marketed, as a means for improving your cholesterol numbers. It's such a simple story. And yet it's wrong on so many accounts."

— Dr. Dwight Lundell

In the introduction I cited a January 2009 study that was published in the *American Heart Journal*. It examined the cholesterol levels of 136,905 patients admitted to the hospital for a cardiovascular event between 2000 and 2006. It found that nearly 75 percent of them had LDL within the "healthy" range, and close to half of them had "optimal" levels below 100 mg/dL. Additionally, over half the patients also had low levels of HDL cholesterol (the so-called "good cholesterol"), which is considered a bad sign. Now isn't that interesting? All the leading health groups are telling us that heart health depends on getting LDL levels lower and lower, and yet the heart attack patients in this study had what is considered healthy levels. So why are we still vilifying LDL?

One big reason is money. You can't miss the radio and TV ads touting the cholesterol-lowering wonder drugs known as statins. What the ads don't mention are the millions of dollars the pharmaceutical companies are spending to deviously market these drugs to the public, and not only through advertising. Doctors and hospitals are given incentives, financial and otherwise, to push statins on us; the most popular of the drugs—Lipitor, Crestor, and Zocor—are huge moneymakers for everyone involved in prescribing them to you.

MOMENT OF CLARITY: "The financial success of the statin drugs to reduce cholesterol deeply embedded this notion of lowering cholesterol levels as a primary means of treating heart disease. Unfortunately, 98 percent of my fellow cardiologists have jumped on this bandwagon. It's enormously profitable and it's paid for many glorious vacations in Orlando and a lot of nice dinners. It's paid for many things for those who promote statins. We're talking about a $29 billion annual industry, so this has fueled a very successful campaign to treat cholesterol. It also took us down this dead end where it has made us stupid about how heart disease was caused."

– Dr. William Davis

MOMENT OF CLARITY: "Taking a statin drug is easy and it kind of pushes the problem away. Also, it does lower something and people like seeing things they can measure go down. And when it does drop, you can be congratulated for a job well done. There are some days that I think if humanity has decided to be this stupid, then I give up."

– Dr. Malcolm Kendrick

Here's a reality check for people who are taking a statin drug: These drugs *will* artificially lower your cholesterol levels, but they will *not* prevent a heart attack, stroke, or cardiovascular disease. Statins can also cause a fairly long list of risky side effects (more on this in the next chapter). And yet, your doctor's first recommendation if you have an elevated cholesterol level is more likely than not a medication. In fact, some doctors recommend everyone take a statin drug and have even pushed for it to put it in our water supply! If changes in diet and lifestyle are even mentioned by your doctor, they will almost invariably be suggested in conjunction with a statin. Doesn't this seem odd to you? Why aren't more physicians thinking beyond prescriptions and questioning an approach that clearly isn't working?

MOMENT OF CLARITY: "There's a definite sense that a change in thinking about cholesterol is under way because quite prominent doctors and even cardiologists and other health professionals are going public with their opposition to the traditional theory. It's seems there are more questions being asked about these things now than ever before. I don't think cholesterol theory will suddenly disappear, because while there's money to be made, I think there's always going to be stout support for it. However, questions are at least being asked, and the Internet is now a rich source of opinion and science, which counters the cholesterol hypothesis. The whole area has opened up and it has allowed much more healthy skepticism about the information we have been given. Overall, I'm optimistic that we're slowly but surely getting to the truth, and that people are benefiting as a result."

– Dr. John Briffa

Doctors Deserve Our Respect, But They Have Been Misled on Cholesterol

Don't get me wrong. I honestly believe that most members of the medical and health profession mean no harm to their patients. I have great respect for doctors, nurses, and registered dietitians. The problem is when the education they are given isn't up-to-date with the latest science and understanding. The intense demands of working long hours or maybe even simple laziness can lead many of these health professionals to put continuing health education on the back-burner once they begin practicing. As a result, they fall back on decades-old science, and this is detrimental to their patients and clients. This is exactly what happened with cholesterol and its supposed role in heart disease.

MOMENT OF CLARITY: "My impression is that most medical practitioners just don't get it; they've been buffaloed by representatives from the pharmaceutical companies, who pass their literature off as scientific education. This makes it very, very difficult for them to make a reasonable assessment of what's really going on with their patients."

– Dr. Philip Blair

Swedish physician and researcher Dr. Uffe Ravnskov (another of the experts featured in this book) was so frustrated by the lack of solid science supporting the cholesterol hypothesis that, in 2001, he formed the International Network of Cholesterol Skeptics (THINCS). The group is composed of respected and like-minded scientists, physicians, academics, and science writers from around the world, all of whom challenge the notion that high cholesterol plays any role in cardiovascular disease.

"Very quickly I realized that we should inform our colleagues and the public about the fraudulent misinformation we have received for many years, and this gave me the idea to create THINCS and its website in 2001," Dr. Ravnskov told me in an interview for this book. As of 2013, one hundred professors, experienced researchers, and journalists have joined the group, in addition to a few anonymous members. In general, the anonymous members choose not to reveal their identity as THINCS supporters out of fear of a loss of research funding. This illustrates just how tough it is to go against the establishment's views, no matter how outdated the information is.

MOMENT OF CLARITY: "A paradigm shift away from the cholesterol hypothesis will not likely occur until the current professors have died or retired."

– Dr. Uffe Ravnskov

Cholesterol Levels and Heart Disease Rates Show No Correlation

One of the major players in THINCS is a Scottish physician named Dr. Malcolm Kendrick, author of the brilliant YouTube video "Cholesterol and

Heart Disease" (http://youtu.be/i8SSCNaaDcE), which graphically disproves—in just seventy-eight seconds!—the cholesterol-heart hypothesis data from the World Health Organization's multinational Monitoring of Trends in Cardiovascular Disease (MONICA). Among other things, the video reveals that Australian aboriginals have the highest rates of heart disease but the lowest levels of cholesterol, while the Swiss, with the highest levels of cholesterol in the world, have just one-third the heart disease of people in the United Kingdom.

MOMENT OF CLARITY: "There is absolutely no correlation between saturated fat intake, cholesterol levels, and heart disease. The most accurate research looking at this issue in different countries is the MONICA (Monitoring of Trends and Determinants in Cardiovascular Disease) study that started in the mid-1980s and is run by the World Health Organization. If you look at the figures, it's extremely clear that the countries whose populations have the highest saturated fat intake tend to have slightly higher cholesterol levels, but all have lower rates of heart disease. We're talking about a difference of 700 percent! The country whose people eat the highest level of saturated fat in Europe is France. Their average total cholesterol is 215 mg/dL, and yet their rate of heart disease is one-seventh that of people in Ukraine, where people eat less than half the amount of saturated fat and their average cholesterol levels are slightly lower. So from this data we learn that the countries with the highest saturated fat consumption all have lower heart disease levels than the countries with the lowest saturated fat consumption. Cholesterol levels vary from around 195–225 mg/dL, with Switzerland having the highest cholesterol average at 250 mg/dL—and the rate of heart disease among the Swiss is the second lowest in Europe and one-fourth of that in the United States."

— Dr. Malcolm Kendrick

In his book *The Cholesterol Myths*, Dr. Ravnskov noted that before statin drugs came along there were more than forty research trials conducted to test whether lowering cholesterol levels would prevent heart attacks. The results were mixed; some showed that fatal heart attacks dropped, while others found that fatal heart attacks went up. When all these studies were combined, the data revealed that as many people died in the group treated to lower cholesterol as died in the untreated control group. Nevertheless, when it was discovered that money could be made selling cholesterol-lowering medications like statins, research like this was quickly quashed. As my UK-based friend Justin Smith (the man behind the must-see documentary *$TATIN NATION*) says, pharmaceutical companies and the medical community suddenly had "$29 billion" reasons to keep quiet. That silence remains deafening today.

MOMENT OF CLARITY: "The statin drugs that people are taking to lower their cholesterol levels actually cause the liver cells to die. When enough liver cells die, there's less cholesterol in the blood. So naturally the cholesterol level goes down. But it's all a big farce!"

– Dr. Fred Kummerow

With evidence mounting against the role of cholesterol in heart disease, more and more independent-thinking physicians and health experts are starting to oppose what is still described as a "hypothesis" or "theory." It is sad and unfortunate that people have dogmatically latched on to the cholesterol-heart theory, treating it as proven fact when unimpeachable data to support it does not exist. People deserve an honest answer, and they deserve it now. In the next chapter we'll delve into the clever marketing of these cholesterol-lowering statin drugs, as well as their demonstrably devastating side effects.

MOMENT OF CLARITY: "In terms of heart health, cholesterol testing is 99 percent irrelevant because cholesterol is not what causes heart disease. Therefore, who cares what your cholesterol level is? It is associated with heart disease but not the primary causal factor."

– Dr. Dwight Lundell

DOCTOR'S NOTE FROM DR. ERIC WESTMAN: Because we have taught this cholesterol hypothesis for years, as if it were the correct explanation for cardiovascular disease, most health professionals are going to believe that it is true. There is a saying that most doctors practice medicine the way they were taught in medical school. We need to educate practicing health professionals through meetings and continuing medical education programs.

KEY CHOLESTEROL CLARITY CONCEPTS

→ Doctors who subscribe to the cholesterol-heart hypothesis are treating patients with decades-old science.

→ Most heart attack victims have "normal" cholesterol levels.

→ There is no correlation between high cholesterol levels and increased heart disease.

→ Statin drugs have become the first treatment option for high cholesterol.

→ Before the introduction of statins, research findings on the correlation between lowering cholesterol and preventing heart attacks were mixed.

→ Many physicians are becoming skeptical of the cholesterol hypothesis.

→ We, as patients, must question health authorities pushing the cholesterol hypothesis.

Chapter 5

Statin Drugs: Magic Pill or Marketed Poison?

MOMENT OF CLARITY: "Before statins, there was really nothing that would lower cholesterol very much—10–15 percent maybe. But with statins you could knock cholesterol down around 30–40 percent. So if you can argue that an elevated cholesterol level causes coronary disease, you've got a big reason why there is now a multi-billion dollar industry."

— Dr. Donald Miller

Technology development in the last couple of decades has been both exciting and awe-inspiring. In that time, we've seen the birth of YouTube, Facebook, Twitter, iPods, iPhones, iPads, Bluetooth, USB ports, X-Box, Wii, and the Segway. All these cool new gadgets and technological advances have their downsides, for sure, but they are more beneficial than harmful. Wouldn't it be nice if that were also true for medical and pharmaceutical developments? In the mid-1990s, Pfizer Pharmaceuticals introduced the cholesterol-lowering statin drug Lipitor (atorvastatin). It hit the marketplace with a bang, quickly becoming the most profitable and best-selling drug in the history of the world.

MOMENT OF CLARITY: "To believe that statin medication is the answer to everything, despite reports that these drugs haven't done much in terms of saving people's lives, is misguided. There's a lot of evidence that supports the fact that you don't need to be on a statin medication."

— Dr. Fred Pescatore

Based on the billions of dollars in annual revenue generated by what so many people describe as magic pills for heart health, other drug companies quickly jumped on the statin bandwagon, including AstraZeneca, which introduced Crestor (rosuvastatin), and Merck, which gave us Zocor (simvastatin). Everybody in the pharmaceutical industry wanted a proverbial piece of the pie. Almost everyone today has a friend or family member (maybe even you!) on one of these supposedly heart-healthy medications. I used to be one of those people.

MOMENT OF CLARITY: "If we lump a bunch of people together who are at particularly high risk for one illness or another and we give them statin drugs, there will be benefits. They're not huge, but there will be benefits. And yet it's not the cholesterol-lowering effects that are providing these benefits. They've been focusing on the wrong lens through which to view heart disease."

– Dr. William Davis

Don't Just Take It from Me: Take It from All These People Who Were Prescribed Statins

Before my 180-pound weight loss success in 2004, my doctor prescribed Lipitor for my high cholesterol. At the time, I was morbidly obese and my total cholesterol levels were 230, which he described to me as dangerously high simply because they were above 200. I can assure you that millions of other people with similar levels have been told the exact same thing, and most doctors automatically prescribe a statin drug as the first line of defense in bringing these cholesterol levels down.

But riddle me this, Batman: Is someone with a total cholesterol of 201 at greater risk of having a heart attack than a someone with a total cholesterol of 199? It's a question few doctors or health practitioners bother to discuss with patients. Most people wouldn't ask anyway; they just obediently do what their doctor tells them to do. That's right: We'll obediently take a medication we know nothing about—a drug that could quite possibly be doing more harm than good.

MOMENT OF CLARITY: "Humans are inherently lazy. That's a simple fact of evolution. We would rather take a shortcut when it appears to be the easier way. Of course, we know that in the vast majority of cases a few diet and exercise changes can have far more profound effects in lowering heart-health risks than could ever be achieved using statins—with nothing but desirable side effects."

– Mark Sisson

Let me introduce you to six people who were advised by their doctors to take statins. See if you can relate to any or all of them:

Nick P. is a forty-nine-year old man from Orlando, Florida with a total cholesterol of 268. His LDL is 164, HDL is 72, and triglycerides (a blood lipid) are 53. Nick's doctor started pushing statins on him long before his numbers reached this level; he had what the doctor called hypercholesterolemia, a dastardly sounding condition that simply means a patient's cholesterol levels are higher than what "authorities" have established as optimal. Bear in mind that high cholesterol in itself is not a disease, and yet Nick's doctor insisted that taking a statin helps people "live longer and healthier" lives.

Cheryl F. is a fifty-nine-year old woman from Carlsbad, California with total cholesterol of 255. Her LDL is 181, HDL is 58, and triglycerides are 80. When she got her cholesterol test results back from her doctor, Cheryl said there was no discussion about why her numbers were supposedly poor and whether changing her diet and lifestyle would help improve her numbers. Her doctor simply wrote a prescription for a statin with no further comment. Interestingly, when she refused to take the statin, Cheryl got a prerecorded telephone call from her health insurance company; they advised her to follow the advice of her doctor as soon as possible, adding that it was critical to her health. They followed up again with a letter stating that high LDL alone causes heart disease, and backed it up with a full-color "educational" newsletter that included an illustration of an artery filled with plaque. Again, this was not the doctor following up; it was the insurance company marketing fear and misinformation in an effort to make more money off the ignorance of patients.

Bob H. is a sixty-nine-year old man from Harrison, Arkansas who started taking 10 mg Lipitor in 2004 on the advice of his doctor. Each year the dosage was upped, reaching 40 mg by 2007. After experiencing a significant increase in joint and muscle pain, Bob went off the drug in 2012. When he told his doctor, the immediate reaction was disappointment. Bob had his cholesterol tested again in early 2013 and the total was 215. The nurse at his doctor's office recommended that he go back on a low-dose statin. When Bob refused and asked his doctor why he kept pushing a medication that brought pain to his body, the doctor said that if he didn't follow the protocol of prescribing statin drugs for people with elevated cholesterol levels, he would be penalized by the medical board. Interesting.

Erin S. is a fifty-five-year old woman from Flagstaff, Arizona with total cholesterol of 251. Her LDL is 160, HDL is 78, and triglycerides are 65. After she got her test results back, the nurse-practitioner asked Erin to come in for a "discussion" about her numbers. When the nurse expressed concern, Erin requested particle-size testing (which we'll discuss in chapter 9), which would provide a direct measurement of her cholesterol. This time, her total cholesterol came back 217, with LDL 145, HDL 71, and triglycerides 42. Her LDL particles were the big and fluffy Pattern A variety, which are considered good, rather than the smaller, denser Pattern B particles, which are considered bad. (Again, don't worry about the terminology; LDL particles will be explained soon). Nevertheless, the nurse counseled that to prevent a heart attack, Erin must immediately begin taking a statin drug. Because she had educated herself, Erin refused. But a seed of doubt planted by a doctor or nurse is a powerful thing, and most people aren't as confident as Erin.

David P. is a twenty-two-year old man from Kennesaw, Georgia with a total cholesterol of 204. His LDL is 138, HDL 56, and triglycerides 52. This young man was chided by the overweight nurse at his doctor's office for his "high" cholesterol test results, and told that the doctor would prescribe a statin drug if he did not switch to a low-fat diet with "lots of vegetables, healthy whole grains, fruits, and lean meats." Once again, fat and cholesterol were targeted as the villains, and statins promoted as the ultimate cure.

Dottie W. is a fifty-five-year old woman from Lexington, Kentucky with total cholesterol of 240. Her LDL is 155, HDL 65 and triglycerides 98. Dottie had already been diagnosed with high cholesterol many years before and prescribed Lipitor by her doctor. She never took it because her other numbers were right where they needed to be. Her doctor kept insisting that she take a statin drug, and when she asked him if he could run a more advanced cholesterol screening, he explained that such a test is only for people with a family history of heart disease and it would not be covered by her health insurance. Not knowing any better, she didn't have it run. One week later, Dottie received a telephone call from her doctor's office, again pushing Lipitor, this time because she has a "family history of high cholesterol." Needless to say, such pressure left Dottie feeling extremely frustrated and angry.

MOMENT "Treating cholesterol with statins is like waving the smoke away
OF CLARITY: from the fire and thinking that you've put it out."

– Dr. Dwight Lundell

Why Have Statin Drugs Become the First Line of Defense against High Cholesterol?

The ubiquity of statin drugs in America today is disturbing. There are certainly people who could stand to benefit from these medications—people who have exhausted smarter and more natural options first, such as changes in diet and lifestyle. But statins have become a doctor's first line of defense; the best resort, not the last resort. And this is despite the fact that these drugs, while being touted as a grand cure-all, have done nothing to stop the rise of heart disease in this country: It is still the number-one killer among both men and women in the United States and it is expected to become a worldwide epidemic by 2020. Instead of prescribing an artificial way to make cholesterol numbers merely look good on paper, maybe doctors and medical researchers should start paying attention to the underlying reasons why cholesterol numbers go up in the first place and what implications that is having on the health of their patients.

MOMENT "Statin drugs unnaturally lower cholesterol without addressing
OF CLARITY: the underlying cause for what caused the elevation in the first
place. Elevated cholesterol can be a symptom of inflammation and it's the cause
of that inflammation that is the root cause of heart disease. This is the essence
of the message I teach my clients. Cholesterol increases to address any damage
that is going on in the blood vessels. Having high cholesterol shouldn't be alarm-
ing, but it should force you to closely examine what is going on."

– Cassie Bjork

A March 2013 study by Cornell University researchers published in the *Journal of General Internal Medicine* found television advertisements of statin medications may be the driving force behind the overprescribing of statin drug therapy and the increase in the diagnosis of patients with high cholesterol. Think about that for a moment. If you see a commercial that tells you that your risk of heart attack or stroke is reduced by taking a cholesterol-lowering drug, and then you get test results that say your cholesterol levels are high, wouldn't your natural response be to agree to take such a drug? Let's not kid ourselves here; they want you to ask your doctor about these drugs because the pharmaceutical companies have sent their good-looking, nicely-dressed reps in to convince them too! This kind of subliminal brainwashing is the purpose of the direct-to-consumer marketing of pharmaceutical drugs like statins. And here's the irony: We don't allow cigarette companies to advertise on TV because cigarettes have been proven to cause illness and death (which, of course, I don't dispute), but we *do* allow pharmaceutical companies to promote drugs that are well-known to cause serious, even life-threatening side effects. If that seems crazy to you, you're not alone.

MOMENT OF CLARITY: "Most people don't realize that statins don't simply block production of cholesterol. They ultimately cause LDL receptors to incorporate the LDL into the cells. And if your LDL receptors aren't working properly, then the statins don't work well."

– Dr. David Diamond

The Wildly Underreported Side Effects of Statin Drugs

When I was taking Lipitor in the early 2000s, I suffered from extreme fatigue, foggy memory, joint and muscle pain, and a lack of mental acuity. On an afternoon in early 2004, I was playing a pickup game of basketball at my church; I went up for a rebound and felt a pain in my thumb—the worst I'd ever experienced. My hand swelled up enough that I drove myself to the emergency room. The doctor said I had a deep tissue bruise. All I had done was grab the rebound in a basketball game, which I had done many times before. But the joints in my fingers had degenerated to such a degree that gripping a ball injured me. Based on what I know now, I'm convinced that wouldn't have happened if I hadn't been taking a statin drug.

When I complained to my primary care physician, who had prescribed Lipitor, he said he would switch me over to a "better" drug, Crestor. I continued to experience many of the same issues because, well, it was just another statin drug. I should point out that I had already lost one hundred pounds, and I continued to lose more in 2004. So after months, I decided to kick the statins. Good riddance! I've been off these medications for nearly a decade and I swear I can still feel their effects in my joints.

MOMENT OF CLARITY: "There are some negative study results about statin drugs that are not being reported to the public. So you now have a bias in the medical literature that touts all the positive results of taking statin medications. The interpretation of this by medical doctors is that prescribing these drugs is okay. It's the wrong answer. Based on the side effects we have seen and the fundamental metabolic pathways that are interrupted by these statin drugs, probably 100 percent of people taking them experience side effects, they just might not be aware of them yet. We know that statins are disrupting their metabolism and negative things are going on. It's just that the these things could take years to manifest."

– Dr. Philip Blair

One of my blog readers alerted me to a dangerous trend in October 2012: Pharmaceutical companies were shifting the focus of their statin marketing from medical doctors (mission accomplished—most of them are convinced of the drugs' benefits) to health insurance companies. Now they, too, are targeting their customers with cholesterol hypothesis "education." In the September 2012 edition of Blue Cross Blue Shield of Illinois's *Blue Vision* monthly employee group newsletter, the company literally gushed over the benefits and safety of statin drugs. The newsletter noted that having "less cholesterol in your blood" lowers "your risk of heart disease, heart attacks, and strokes." The article added that you *need* a statin drug to drop LDL, which was erroneously described as the "amount of cholesterol fat circulating in your blood that often is deposited in the artery walls."

The information contained in this newsletter was incredibly misleading. But coming as it does from a respected health insurance company, is it surprising that those who don't know the truth might follow this advice? The thing that struck me the most was the statement that "statins are safe," as if they are risk-free. Yes, Blue Cross Blue Shield of Illinois did admit to some side effects, but "the benefits of taking a statin outweigh the chance of problems."

Here's one big reason why Blue Cross can't possibly know that: The side effects have never been thoroughly researched. Although I have heard the claim that only 5 percent of people taking statins have serious problems with them, there are an overwhelming number of complaints on online forums, such as *Taking Lipitor and Hate It*, which include some truly horrific anecdotes. And one study of statin drug use, published in the medical journal *Annals of Internal Medicine*, found that 17 percent of 100,000 participants reported having side effects, and two-thirds of that 17 percent elected to stop taking the statins as a result.

MOMENT OF CLARITY: "Statins have several different mechanisms of action in the body that might reduce the risk of heart disease in ways that have nothing to do with cholesterol. For example, statins are anti-inflammatory, and inflammation appears to be a key underlying process in the development of cardiovascular disease. There is a current vogue for doctors to treat people's cholesterol down to a particular level, but this approach has never actually been tested for its effectiveness. In fact, in people without a history of heart disease or stroke, maybe a hundred people need to be treated to prevent one heart attack. That's great for the person who is saved from a heart attack, but what about the ninety-nine others who do not derive this benefit? And bear in mind, now, that the side effects of statins are quite common, with some estimates putting the risk at about 20 percent. Suddenly, statins are not looking like the wonder drugs they're so often made out to be."

— **Dr. John Briffa**

MOMENT OF CLARITY: "Hundreds of millions of people at this point are compromising their health by taking a statin drug, and it's just horrible."

— **Stephanie Seneff**

MOMENT OF CLARITY: "Statins can integrate themselves into your mitochondria to create defective mitochondria that perpetuate themselves. And so it's almost as if you are introducing a malignancy. This is why people who take these cholesterol-lowering medications tend to have such devastating effects on their health, even long after they stop taking them."

— **Dr. Philip Blair**

I consider myself very fortunate: My statin side effects were confined to a few aches and pains. But for NASA astronaut and physician Dr. Duane Graveline, another one of the experts interviewed for and quoted in this book, a nightmare experience resulted in a steady decline in health. Dr. Graveline began taking statins for high cholesterol in March 1999. His total cholesterol during an annual physical had come in at 270 and he believed, like almost all of his medical colleagues, that cholesterol was the cause of heart disease. In fact, when he was in family practice, he had treated his patients with "one cholesterol buster after another, believing cholesterol to be the cause of atherosclerosis." When he began taking 10 mg of Lipitor for his own elevated numbers, there was no mention of any side effects. Dr. Graveline simply went along with what his NASA doctor said about the drugs, and he was excited by the prospect of seeing his cholesterol numbers drop by as much as half.

It took two months for Dr. Graveline to experience his first episode of a rare medical condition known as transient global amnesia (TGA), which impairs new memory formation and causes some retrograde loss of memory. Yes, his total cholesterol had dropped by 115 points just six weeks after he began taking Lipitor, but here he was sitting in an emergency room with a bunch of ER doctors who had never even heard of TGA. It took six hours and a neurologist's exam before Dr. Graveline was able to figure out what was happening to him.

MOMENT OF CLARITY: "The best way to inform people about the problem with statin treatment is to talk about the many serious side effects. When an older patient tells his doctor that he has pain in his muscles, the doctor usually responds that this is a normal effect of aging. The same goes for memory loss. Side effects from drug treatment usually appear immediately, but since several months may pass before they appear after the start of statin treatment, neither the doctor nor the patient realize that the symptoms are due to the drug. But if their symptoms disappear as soon as patients come off these medications, it is impossible to tell them to continue taking statins."

– Dr. Uffe Ravnskov

MOMENT OF CLARITY: "In the early '90s, when people were trying to prove that statins were worthwhile, there was a shocking study where they gave statins to patients who had heart attacks. There was an improvement in long-term mortality, but there was also improvement in the short-term mortality rates—in like the thirty-day range. That didn't make much sense because they didn't have enough time to change their cholesterol metabolism, much less remove all the cholesterol that was in the plaques they already had. It was quite a mystery because it wasn't working by removing cholesterol from plaque. That sort of added to the glamour of statins."

– Dr. Ken Sikaris

Dr. Graveline told the neurologist about the Lipitor he was taking and the curt response was, "Statins do not do this." This brain specialist told his patient to stay on the Lipitor, but Dr. Graveline had become "suspicious" and decided to stop taking the drug while he investigated what had happened to him. He spoke with roughly thirty doctors and pharmacists about the possible relationship between statin drug use and cognitive impairment, and they all told him there was no connection.

A few months later, in March 2000, Dr. Graveline returned to see his NASA physician, who wanted to put him back on Lipitor, this time at half the dose, 5 mg. Dr. Graveline agreed. Two months later he had another episode of TGA, which lasted for twelve hours; he woke up in the ER. After this incident, Dr. Graveline knew his suspicions about statins were justified. He began conducting his own research, to see if anyone else was experiencing similar side effects.

TGA is extremely rare, but most people on statins experience various deleterious cognitive effects, like confusion or disorientation, and too often those symptoms are chalked up to aging. Jokes about memory loss go hand in hand with getting older, but when you think about the tens of millions of people who are taking statins, you have to wonder if we might be laughing at the wrong people. Do the doctors prescribing these drugs know the truth about them and simply choose not to tell their patients, or are they just as clueless as their patients? Either way, it would be ludicrous if it weren't so dangerous.

MOMENT OF CLARITY: "The only patients I recommend statins to are those who refuse to change their diet. That's the role statins can play for a noncompliant patient."

— Dr. Jeffry Gerber

These days Dr. Graveline is warning people about the dangers of statin drugs on his outstanding educational website, SpaceDoc.com. He's also written four books on the subject: *Lipitor, Thief of Memory; Statin Drugs Side Effects; The Statin Damage Crisis;* and *The Dark Side of Statins.* In the last decade, Dr. Graveline has reduced his cholesterol to 200, and he did it naturally, with a low-carb, high-fat diet that includes the regular consumption of whole milk, real butter, and whole eggs. His cognitive decline, which began with TGA, has progressed, however, into amyotrophic lateral sclerosis (ALS), aka Lou Gehrig's disease—a condition he absolutely believes resulted from the statin drugs his doctor prescribed.

Dr. Graveline told me the ALS is "slowly incapacitating" him and that he will "soon be in a wheelchair." It continues to concern him that most people are completely unaware of the "inevitable side effects" of statin drugs, which include interfering with critical brain function. "There is no way these statin drugs can block cholesterol without at the same time blocking such vital biochemicals as CoQ10 and dolichols," Dr. Graveline says. "The effects of cholesterol on memory are fully documented. Cholesterol is vital for both the formation and function of each memory synapse in our brains. As thousands of people can testify, when you have no cholesterol, you have no memory."

He explains that CoQ10 and dolichols (long-chain unsaturated organic compounds) are what the body uses to build mitochondria, which, because they supply cellular energy, are often described as "cellular power plants." If these vital parts of normal body function become depleted, says Dr. Graveline, "damage and mutations result, causing myopathies, neuropathies, hundreds of statin-associated ALS cases, as well as organ damage, such as hepatitis and pancreatitis."

Dr. Graveline says that rates of TGA and ALS have been on the rise since statin drugs were introduced, but few are making the connection. So he is using his own tragic situation to alert people to the serious dangers of cholesterol-lowering medications. Unfortunately, nothing will change until doctors and their patients educate themselves. In the meantime, if you are taking a statin drug or are over the age of fifty, supplement your diet with coenzyme Q10, or CoQ10 for short. A Danish study found that supplementing with CoQ10 can cut mortality by half in patients with heart failure. It's available in any pharmacy and a bit pricey, but the payoff to your health makes it worth every penny.

MOMENT OF CLARITY: "There's evidence that taking statins can increase the risk of cancer and birth defects in animals and decrease cognitive function. But the evidence isn't that strong since all of the attention is being put on those people with high cholesterol9/."

– Dr. Chris Masterjohn

Why Statin Drug Therapy Might Not Be Effective for Women

Entire books could be written debating the necessity of statin drugs, but there's compelling evidence that they are less effective for women than for men. A ten-year study of over 52,000 subjects, conducted by Norwegian researchers and published in the August 2011 issue of the *Journal of Evaluation in Clinical Practice*, showed that women with "high cholesterol" levels (above 270 mg/dL) had close to 30 percent *less* chance of dying of heart disease, a heart attack, or a stroke than those women with normal to low cholesterol (under 193 mg/dL). .

A year earlier, an analysis of eleven randomized, double-blind, placebo-controlled studies was published in the *Archives of Internal Medicine*. It found that women taking statin drugs did not experience the same benefits as men taking the same drugs. In fact, women on statin drugs had a *greater* risk of death by any means (known as "all-cause mortality"), including strokes. The analysis went on to suggest that putting a woman on a statin could potentially be putting her at greater risk of cardiovascular issues by unnecessarily lowering her cholesterol levels with a pill. Whoa!

Finally, the results of a randomized clinical trial of more than 1,000 patients, published in the June 2012 issue of *Archives of Internal Medicine*, found that women experienced a disproportionate level of extreme fatigue and decreased energy levels after taking statin medications to lower their cholesterol. So if you are a mother or a career woman taking statins, don't assume it's your busy life that's zapped you of energy; it might be those cholesterol pills prescribed to supposedly make you healthier. At the very least, all these studies make it clear that it's not only worth taking a closer look at the evidence, it's worth asking if women should be lowering their cholesterol at all.

Should *Anyone* Be Taking a Statin Drug?

One of the experts I interviewed for this book is a highly respected lipidologist named Dr. Thomas Dayspring. Full disclosure: He is on the Speaker's Bureau of the pharmaceutical companies AstraZeneca, Reliant, Abbott, Merck, Schering-Plough, and Sanofi-Aventis, and is a consultant for Abbott and Reliant. He is therefore not adverse to statins and he falls into the camp that thinks side effects are minimal. But even he believes that lifestyle should be the first step to improving heart health and cholesterol numbers. "Most of the time, changes in your diet and lifestyle can be huge," Dr. Dayspring said in an interview for this book. "The biggest problem with telling people to change their diet and lifestyle is that everybody thinks that means going on a low-fat diet. But it is critical to get with a doctor who has up-to-date knowledge regarding what a healthy lifestyle actually means and not necessarily what the American Heart Association says in terms of a low-fat diet."

MOMENT OF CLARITY: "I've never really used statins with my patients because I knew the right approach to cholesterol control and the truth about the cholesterol myths has a lot to do with using a low-carbohydrate diet. If we can get people on the right kind of diet, then their risk of heart disease is substantially reduced. And that's what we're talking about here—improving the cardiometabolic risk, not cholesterol. Unfortunately, both the lay public and the medical practitioners have had it ingrained in them that somehow cholesterol is negatively involved in heart health, but nothing could be further from the truth."

— Dr. Philip Blair

We'll be discussing the most up-to-date nutritional information later. Just know that people who decide to ditch statins and try to manage their heart health through diet and lifestyle have to be incredibly vigilant and methodical about what they are doing. "The real problem with most people is that they just don't do what's required to see improvements happen," said Dr. Dayspring. "If you want to go totally drug-free, then you have to get serious about lifestyle and diet changes."

MOMENT OF CLARITY: "My husband was put on a high-dose statin in 2007 and that is what started me on this journey. I began to educate myself, and he started to implement a lot of the things that I learned. His doctor insisted that he continue taking a statin, but he quit after one year and he's doing great. He was nervous at first about eating cholesterol-rich foods, like eggs, gizzards, and seafood. He was also nervous about doing his cholesterol test after eating those foods. It turned out that his HDL went up and his LDL went down, all as a direct result of the extra cholesterol he was getting from his food. If you get it from your food, it doesn't have to end up in the LDL."

— Stephanie Seneff

Researchers have seen correlations between statin drugs and an increased risk of developing diabetes, Alzheimer's disease, and, as Dr. Duane Graveline shared, the depletion of the key nutrient CoQ10. In a study published in the April 2013 issue of the journal *Metabolic Syndrome and Related Disorders*, researchers at Oregon State University showed that statin-induced diabetes occurs as a direct result of CoQ10 depletion. Holy crap!

Isn't it the irony of all ironies that the best drug for lowering cholesterol levels as a means of protecting your cardiovascular health also depletes your body of the natural production of CoQ10, a key heart-health nutrient—as well as a nutrient that decreases your chances of developing adult-onset diabetes? Hmm. Why don't we ever hear the statin drug manufacturers talking about this in their slick television commercials? So much for truth in advertising.

MOMENT OF CLARITY: "People should really want to feel comfortable about what they are doing and realize what the more natural thing to do is. Some people trust technology or what their cardiologist tells them is the right thing to do. Technological advances in medications have become their health god and now they bow down to it as their religion. Meanwhile, others don't trust the changing technology and stick with a more natural, commonsense approach. Know where you stand. Either you stand on the side of nature or you stand on the side of technology. If you fall into the latter group, then you probably won't believe anything negative you hear about statins or cholesterol and you'll spend a lot of money on tests and drugs that will continue to be argued and debated. But if you believe in nature, find a doctor who matches up with your health philosophy. It all comes down to natural versus intervention. The goal is to get people away from dependence on pills and to start eating right. There have been a lot of publications showing that if you have heart failure, you should not take a statin. And no one is paying attention to this. The only people who I would ever recommend going on statins are male smokers who have had a heart attack and won't quit smoking."

– Dr. Cate Shanahan

In May 2007, Dr. Beatrice Golomb, a researcher at the University of California–San Diego, released the results of her independently funded "Statin Effects Study," the first of its kind to examine and compare patient feedback on the effects of these FDA-approved drugs. After sifting through the responses from the over 4,100 participants, Dr. Golomb and her research team found that:

- ▶ Most of the "adverse effects" occur in higher doses of statins.

- ▶ Recurring symptoms happen frequently after the first side effect.

- ▶ Typical reactions to statin drugs include pain in muscles; trouble remembering things; a tingling, burning, or numbing sensation; and a general sense of irritability.

- ▶ Other symptoms include mood changes, violent nightmares, liver and stomach problems, trouble breathing, profuse sweating, weight gain, breast enhancement, dry skin, rash, impotence, and changes in blood pressure.

- ▶ Statins also negatively impact protein in the urine, kidney function, and the heart.

MOMENT OF CLARITY: "You can smoke cigarettes for thirty years before anything goes wrong. People have been taking statins for less than thirty years. But if you look at the underlying metabolic catastrophe that you're wreaking on the body from taking these cholesterol-lowering drugs, it's not a pretty picture. I've seen some significant, really debilitating, and even life-threatening side effects from patients taking statins. And that's just my observations as one doctor, who doesn't work full time. If I'm seeing this many, how many more people are out there are being poisoned and killed by these drugs? I tell patients that statins may add fifteen years to your life, but they don't make you live fifteen years longer. They *will* make you feel fifteen years older."

– Dr. Malcolm Kendrick

The researchers are quick to point out in their analysis that all these symptoms may or may not be directly related to statin drug use; they are simply what the study participants shared regarding their health while taking them. The results of "The Statin Effects Study" have been published in such peer-reviewed journals as *Journal of the American Heart Association*, the *Archives of Internal Medicine, Controlled Clinical Trials*, and *Annals of Internal Medicine*. More importantly, the findings—shared publicly at StatinEffects.info—are available to any physicians prescribing these drugs to their hypercholesterolemic patients. Is the message getting through to these doctors? It doesn't look like it: Statins remain the primary treatment modality for high cholesterol and heart disease prevention.

MOMENT "It's entirely reasonable to try everyone on diet first, although
OF CLARITY: people who have had a coronary event or procedure should be
on statins out the door."

— Dr. Ronald Krauss

Deciding whether you want to take a statin medication to treat your
"high cholesterol" is an issue you should seriously discuss with your doctor.
There is evidence that statins may provide some powerful anti-inflammatory benefits, and maybe they should be marketed as anti-inflammatory medications—especially if, as more and more studies suggest, having higher
cholesterol might be a positive rather than a negative in heart disease risk.

According to a study published in the October 12, 2005 issue of the
Journal of the American Medical Association, the average total cholesterol
levels for people aged twenty to seventy-four fell from 222 to 203 between
1960 and 2002. Healthy total cholesterol levels are assumed to be below 200.
People aged fifty and older were given the credit for bringing this number down significantly; Americans sixty to seventy-four years old saw their
average levels dip from 232 to 204 in men, or a 12 percent drop, and from
263 to 223 for women, or a 15 percent drop. The study authors noted that
statin drug use from 1993 to 2002 nearly tripled from 3.4 percent to 9.3
percent. Interestingly, although total cholesterol levels dropped, triglyceride levels inched upward. In chapter 10 we'll get into why this is not a good
thing.

MOMENT "Cholesterol is not the problem. Cholesterol is one of the most
OF CLARITY: important biochemicals in the human body. Inflammation, not cholesterol, underlies atherosclerosis."

— Dr. Duane Graveline

The bottom line? If you have high cholesterol but have no heart disease
and have never experienced a heart attack, there is no compelling evidence
that you should be taking a statin drug. Indeed, it may do you more harm
than good. Before you take a statin, make sure you have exhausted any and
all natural dietary and lifestyle options. Just keep in mind that even when
it comes to diet, there's a lot of debunking of what we have always believed
is true going on as well. In the next chapter we'll take a look at the typical

"heart-healthy" nutritional advice and how that advice, like statin drugs, may be doing us more harm than good.

MOMENT OF CLARITY: "If you look at the recommendations on the statins, it doesn't say that high cholesterol alone is justification for taking these drugs. Too often people only have high cholesterol and the doctor will automatically prescribe a statin without any other component of metabolic syndrome or any heart disease risk factor being present."

— Dr. David Diamond

DOCTOR'S NOTE FROM DR. ERIC WESTMAN: I shudder to think that medical education and the current healthcare system has led most doctors to believe that medications are the only effective tools that are available to patients. The cholesterol-heart hypothesis training and the lack of time to do little more than prescribe medications created the perfect environment for this to happen.

KEY CHOLESTEROL CLARITY CONCEPTS

→ **Lowering cholesterol through drugs is a multibillion-dollar industry.**

→ **Statins are pushed on patients with total cholesterol levels over 200.**

→ **Side effects from taking statins are much more prevalent than is commonly believed.**

→ **Pharmaceutical companies target insurance companies with the message that statins promote heart health.**

→ **Studies have shown certain common side effects among statin users.**

Chapter 6

What Does *Heart Healthy* Really Mean?

MOMENT OF CLARITY: "One of the most perverse things about cholesterol is this: I can guarantee that I can lower your LDL readings and your total cholesterol readings by giving you a great big dose of omega-6 fats. I can give you exactly the wrong thing for your heart health to lower the numbers. Your blood cholesterol levels will drop like a stone. You'll drop your levels by 13–18 percent and your doctor will be happy with your progress. But what you've done to your body is probably the absolute worst thing you could ever do."

— David Gillespie

Consider the simple phrase *heart healthy*. What does that actually mean to you? We can all probably agree on "heart-healthy" actions: no smoking, regular physical activity, keeping blood pressure at normal levels, and maintaining a healthy weight. But can we agree on the best possible diet? We see the words *heart healthy* plastered across the front packaging and gobble up those foods, assuming they will keep our hearts ticking longer. But do they?

MOMENT OF CLARITY: "The endgame, of course, is not to have a heart attack, sudden cardiac death, three stents, or bypass surgery. What we're really talking about here is trying to put a stop to, prevent, and avert coronary disease and atherosclerosis. I think we have to ask how people develop coronary atherosclerosis. The problem is there's not just one reason, there's a whole long list of over three hundred causes. But we don't have to consider all three hundred because many of them overlap to an incredible degree."

— Dr. William Davis

Let's take a quick test. Which of the following foods do you consider "heart healthy"?

- Oatmeal

- Roasted nuts

- Egg whites

- Canola, corn, safflower, peanut, sesame, soybean, and sunflower oils

- Nonstick vegetable oil spray (like Pam)

- Fat-free cheese

- Fruits

- Skim milk or soy milk

- Beans

- Margarine (I Can't Believe It's Not Butter, Benecol, or Smart Balance)

- Whole-grain pasta

- Low-fat yogurt

- Brown rice

- Fat-free crackers and chips

- Chicken breast and other lean meats

- Vegetables

- Fat-free or light salad dressings

- Whole-grain breads and cereals

- Fruit juice

- Tofu

Now look at this next list. Do you consider any of these foods to be "heart-healthy"?

- Bacon
- Whole eggs
- Butter
- Salmon
- Lard
- Coconut
- Avocado
- Full-fat sour cream
- Full-fat milk and cheese
- Fatty cuts of beef or poultry
- Pork
- Coconut, avocado, and macadamia nut oils
- Raw nuts
- Nut butters like almond, macadamia, and hazelnut
- Full-fat cream cheese
- Dark chocolate
- Cream
- Fish oil
- Green leafy, nonstarchy vegetables
- Organ meats

If you're like most Americans, you probably consider the first list of foods "heart-healthy" and the second list anything but. Guess what? The very opposite is true. Doctors, nutritionists, and health gurus have been proclaiming the amazing health benefits of low-fat and low-cholesterol diets for decades, so it wouldn't surprise me if you think I've finally gone too far. But, once again, the evidence is piling up against what conventional wisdom has been telling us for decades.

DOCTOR'S NOTE FROM DR. ERIC WESTMAN: We are in the
   midst of what is called a paradigm shift—otherwise known
   as a fundamental change in thinking. There was a time
   when most people thought the sun went around the earth.
   In fact, if you look at the sun's motion during the day, it
   certainly appears as if the sun is going around the earth. This
   was known as the "geocentric" model of the universe (geo
   is derived from the Greek word for "earth"). It took many
   astronomers making detailed observations of the night sky to
   figure out that there were other planets and that the earth
   actually went around the sun. This is now known as the
   "heliocentric" model of the universe (helio is derived from the
   Greek word for "sun"). In a similar way, when you look at
   the arteries that are diseased with atherosclerosis (hardening
   of the arteries), there is fat in them. So it would make sense
   that the fat in the diet would lead to the fat in the arteries
   (the dietary fat hypothesis of heart disease). However, we can
   now examine in greater detail the particles that are carrying
   the fat into the arteries—the small LDL cholesterol particles
   that come from the VLDL (very low-density lipoprotein)
   cholesterol particles, which come from the liver. And where
   does the fat from the liver come from? From dietary
   carbohydrates! So there is a paradigm shift occurring from
   the "dietary fat hypothesis" to the "dietary carbohydrate
   hypothesis" of heart disease.

MOMENT OF CLARITY: "In dietetics school I was taught that cholesterol and saturated fat cause heart disease. And I'm still seeing this same message being taught to new registered dietitians. Furthermore, I was taught that the treatment for heart disease is to eat a high-grain diet, especially the complex carbs, low-fat, and low cholesterol. That means no butter, no eggs, and teaching people to eat cereal or oatmeal for breakfast every morning. The goal was to get as much cholesterol and saturated fat out of the diet as possible."

– Cassie Bjork

All the foods on the first list have a few things in common: They are either low in fat and cholesterol or high in carbohydrates. The foods on the second list are high in fat and generally lower in carbs. If you accept the theory that eating more "fatty" foods will raise your LDL and total cholesterol levels—and, thus, increase your risk of heart disease, heart attack, or stroke—then you would choose foods from the first list. It all sounds perfectly logical, right? Well …

MOMENT OF CLARITY: "One of the problems with the cholesterol message is that it has become a part of conventional thinking. You hear it all the time—on television commercials and even in television shows—that consuming cholesterol-rich foods like eggs is causing harm to heart health. And you look at a product like Cheerios being marketed as cholesterol-lowering. So, culturally, it's a way of thinking that cholesterol is somehow toxic and you want to have as little cholesterol in your body and in your mouth as possible. It's also perpetuated by all these diet gurus connecting elevated cholesterol levels in the blood to your consumption of saturated fat. Our entire society has accepted this mistaken notion that cholesterol and saturated fat are toxic. And of course, animal-based foods contain these two agents in high quantities, so that's why the vegetarian diet is believed to be healthy."

– Dr. David Diamond

Heart Healthy Is Code for Eating Less Fat and More Carbohydrates

If we start looking at this "heart-healthy" idea through a new prism—that cholesterol is not the cause of heart disease (just in case you missed it, this is a major theme in *Cholesterol Clarity*)—then perpetuating the idea that eating low-fat, high-carb foods like the ones in that first list becomes seriously wrong, even detrimental to our health. And that brings up the million-dollar question very few people even bother to ask: What exactly are the unintended consequences to heart health of eating less fat and more carbohydrates? This is the critical point in our next chapter. But for the sake of argument, I'm going to ask you to accept for the moment that cutting down on fat and eating more "healthy" whole grains might actually increase your risk of heart disease.

MOMENT OF CLARITY: "We have had great success in Sweden informing the population—in stories in the newspapers and in the popular medical magazines—of the bad dietary advice they have received from the authorities. Most Swedish people today know that saturated fat is not bad and that the devil's name is carbohydrates. In fact, every now and then butter is sold out in the grocery stores."

— Dr. Uffe Ravnskov

MOMENT OF CLARITY: "My advice is never believe anything you see in the media about medical stuff."

— Dr. Dwight Lundell

The Incorrect "Heart-Healthy" Message Invades Popular Culture

In America, the low-fat, high-carb message has become so deeply in"grain"ed (pardon the pun) that it seeps into nearly every corner of our culture—even TV sitcoms. To relax, my wife Christine and I enjoy watching popular television comedies. And even *they* perpetuate the "heart-healthy" propaganda! Take the recently canceled CBS comedy *Rules of Engagement*. In one scene, the married characters Audrey and Jeff were sitting in their favorite diner. Jeff wanted to order bacon, eggs, and toast with butter. But when the waitress came over, Audrey—in response to a "high cholesterol" diagnosis from Jeff's doctor—orders her husband a "healthier" meal of egg whites, dry toast, and turkey bacon.

MOMENT OF CLARITY: "Without question, cholesterol and saturated fat are the Siamese twins of the anticholesterol campaign, joined at the hip and forever demonized, despite several major studies just in the past few years showing that saturated fat has *nothing* to do with heart disease."

— Dr. Jonny Bowden

Here's another example, also on CBS: Whenever the overweight couple on the sitcom *Mike and Molly* try to lose weight and get healthy, it's always about cutting back on portion size and calories; they end up eating foods that are disgusting to them, and, in general, make themselves miserable. In

fact, late-night host David Letterman—who famously had a total cholesterol level of 680 and emergency quintuple heart bypass surgery in 2000—
contributed his two cents in one of his famous "Top Ten" lists: "Top Ten
Signs You're Watching Too Much Television." At number nine, Letterman
exclaimed, "You lie awake at night worrying about Mike and Molly's cholesterol."

Speaking of Letterman, he was relentless in targeting New Jersey Governor Chris Christie during the GOP convention in 2012. In one segment
he joked that there was a "Chris Christie Cholesterol Clock" marking the
obese governor's rising cholesterol levels. "Yikes!" Letterman exclaimed at
one point, "If things remain the same, it should pass the national debt by
October."

Scenes and jokes like these perpetuate the incorrect notion that eating
fat makes you fat, raises your cholesterol, and puts you on a one-way road
to heart disease.

MOMENT OF CLARITY: "Saturated fats are natural fats and the body prefers them as an energy source."

— Dr. Jeffry Gerber

Did anyone bother to ask David Letterman why his total cholesterol got
to be 680 despite the fact that he's *never* been fat? And if obesity doesn't lead
to higher cholesterol and heart disease or the need for emergency coronary
bypass surgery, then what does? Surely there's more to this story than what
we've been told. And there is. In chapter 7 we look at the failure of the low-
fat message, and why a high-fat, low-carb nutritional approach might be
more heart-healthy than you think. You read that right: A *high-fat* diet is
heart healthy! Stay tuned.

MOMENT OF CLARITY: "People have tried to make lifestyle changes before and they've failed because they are using the ones the medical profession have long touted. They say you need to eat low-fat, high-carb, and exercise more. The implication is that if you don't do these things, then you are stupid, lazy, or uncommitted. We need to throw that thinking out. People would like to be en-gaged, but they are totally frustrated by the lack of results and the impossibility of good changes happening from these traditional ways. When people are frustrated with these things, they turn to themselves and say, 'It must be me. I'm a failure.

I have a problem.' But, in reality, a low-fat, low-calorie program fails because of the incredible hunger it induces and the metabolic disruption that occurs. So these people are prone to failure, but they manifest these serious diseases. Finally, when people realize they are desperate and getting worse, they look for an alternative. That's when the door opens and we find patients receptive to a low-carbohydrate lifestyle change that works. We monitor them, hold them accountable, and give them the details they need to have in order to be successful. That's why we have gotten 90 percent positive results."

— Dr. Philip Blair

DOCTOR'S NOTE FROM DR. ERIC WESTMAN: Don't pay attention to the labeling of the foods in terms of being 'heart-healthy.' We teach people to mainly eat foods that don't have labels at all.

KEY CHOLESTEROL CLARITY CONCEPTS

→ **A heart-healthy eating regimen is assumed to be a low-fat, high-carb diet.**

→ **Cutting fat and eating more whole grains may not protect your heart.**

→ **Even popular culture perpetuates the misguided low-fat, low-cholesterol message.**

→ **Fat doesn't make you fat, nor is it to blame for heart disease.**

Chapter 7

Why Low Fat Ain't All That

MOMENT OF CLARITY: "Most doctors don't know anything about nutrition. In terms of nutritional counseling, many of my patients want to be referred to a nutritionist or a registered dietitian. Unless you have diabetes, no insurance company is going to pay for it. Then, the majority of RDs are giving the standard high-carb, low-fat diet advice. That is the absolute opposite of what most patients need to be doing. So it's a vicious cycle going on."

– Dr. Rocky Patel

DOCTOR'S NOTE FROM DR. ERIC WESTMAN: I had a wake-up call when I was at a family reunion and heard about the experience of a relative. His wife was a nurse, and out of well-intentioned concern she mentioned to him that it was common for corporate executives to get exercise treadmill tests to determine any underlying heart disease (coronary artery blockage), whether they had risk factors for heart disease or not. So he decided to have an exercise treadmill test, and it was "positive," meaning that it suggested—but did not prove—that he might have heart disease. He then had a heart catheterization and they found that he had no coronary artery blockage at all—he had gotten a "false positive." This situation happens occasionally and is just accepted as part of the screening process for heart disease, and that didn't bother me. What bothered me was that the hospital dietitian advised him, "Be sure to change your diet to low fat to prevent heart disease." But he didn't have heart disease! I told my cousin that he shouldn't change a thing. After living fifty-some years, he had no trace of coronary *artery disease. For years, American dietitians and doctors have promoted the one-size-fits-all low-fat diet, believing it will fix everything. It will even fix problems that aren't there!*

This may come as a shock to you, but the majority of medical doctors (including probably your family physician) are lucky if they have more than a week or two of nutritional training as part of their medical education. In 2007, when I began interviewing renowned physicians on my podcast, I was astounded to learn of the minuscule role nutrition plays in traditional medical education. And yet our doctors are the ones advising us on the healthiest ways to eat, whether it's cutting down on fat intake, eating more grains, or reducing calories. That would be like your plumber telling you how to fix your lawnmower.

MOMENT OF CLARITY: "Most doctors are misinformed about the role nutrition can play in improving health, and practicing physicians don't have the time to follow the scientific literature themselves."

– Dr. Uffe Ravnskov

MOMENT OF CLARITY: "Physicians are notoriously unfamiliar with nutrition. Many patients could benefit from weight loss, but most doctors don't have the resources, interest, or time to advise them effectively. Nutrition is seen as a weak sibling to drugs and it requires effort to counsel patients to modify eating habits. It's a barrier because it's a much more labor-intensive, less satisfying experience than prescribing a pill that's going to lower the LDL by 40 percent."

– Dr. Ronald Krauss

So where, exactly, did we get the idea that fat is the grand evil cause not only of heart disease, but of many of our physical ailments as well? I alluded to the answer in chapter 1, but here it is in a nutshell: In the 1950s, nutritional health scientist Ancel Keys began investigating why American businessmen were experiencing high rates of heart disease; he surmised that it had something to do with higher cholesterol. Out of this came his infamous Seven Countries Study, which concluded that those nations with diets lower in animal fat had lower rates of heart disease, while those nations with diets higher in animal fat had higher rates of heart disease. The results seemed so neat and clean, and yet it was a totally bogus study.

MOMENT OF CLARITY: "The traditional view of mainstream medicine holds that heart disease, atherosclerosis, and plaque are caused by cholesterol—this has been the main theme of cholesterol science dating back to the days of Ancel Keys and even before that, with the creation of the lipid hypothesis, which stated that eating saturated fat in the diet raises cholesterol, which leads to heart disease. That's the old school of thought. I have graduated from that school and I no longer subscribe to that way of thinking. I tend to think about cholesterol and heart disease in terms of the theory of inflammation and oxidative stress. It is clearly these forces that act on cholesterol and lipoprotein molecules to cause plaque."

– Dr. Jeffry Gerber

Although Keys could have included a total of twenty-two countries in his research data—including countries where people ate more fat with very little heart disease and countries where people ate less fat with more heart disease—he chose to leave those statistics out of his conclusions. They simply didn't fit his theory about saturated fat: that it raises cholesterol levels, which leads to heart disease. Based on the work of Ancel Keys, the American Heart Association, in 1956, officially announced that real foods previously deemed healthy, like butter, lard, eggs, and beef, were now suddenly bad for you; that's when the birth of the low-fat diet movement began in earnest, and it's still the pervading school of thought regarding heart health today. I'm betting that future generations will look back on this era as the truly dark days of nutrition in world history.

MOMENT OF CLARITY: "Superimposed on all this was the work of Ancel Keys and the McGovern Commission, where the low-fat approach became official policy. Keys published his Seven Countries Study and the interesting thing was that he himself publicized the correlation between saturated fat and cholesterol with heart disease. But on page 262 of his study, there's this interesting quote: 'The fact that the incidence of the rate of coronary heart disease significantly correlated with the average percentage of carbohydrates from sucrose in the diet is explained by the intercorrelation of sucrose with saturated fat.' Keys knew that sugar was just as closely correlated with heart disease as fat, but this was buried in the study."

– Dr. Dwight Lundell

Living through the Dark Days of the Low-Fat Diet Fad

The ripple effect that Keys's research would have on consumer choices was profound. Low-fat and fat-free products began flooding the market. My mom grappled with excess weight for most of her life; back in the '80s, when I was a child, she was on one low-fat diet after another. Rice cakes and fat-free ice cream and cookies began filling the food aisles of grocery stores during the Reagan era, and they continue to line those shelves today.

MOMENT OF CLARITY: "There is a huge low-fat food industry that is making billions of dollars worldwide by removing the fat from foods and sticking carbohydrates and sugars in their place. So I think the reasons this information about cholesterol still exists is really all about money."

— Dr. Malcolm Kendrick

The notion that eating saturated fat raises your cholesterol and puts you at greater risk of a heart attack or developing heart disease has led to the growth of at least two major profit machines: Big Pharma and Big Food. Go into any grocery store and look for a food label making a health claim. What you'll likely find are phrases like *naturally fat-free* on a bag of marshmallows or *lower your cholesterol* on a box of Cheerios. What's the clear marketing intention of using these terms? That's right, it gives you permission to eat these foods under the guise that they are "good" for you! Never mind the fact they are mostly highly processed and filled with gobs of sugar, refined grains, and preservatives that contribute more to the development of chronic diseases than the perceived health benefits you get from consuming them.

MOMENT OF CLARITY: "I think greater acceptance of the low-carb message is coming. At the meetings I attend, you see more and more emphasis on the role of carbs in the diet. Don't get me wrong, there's still a lot of really bad information being promulgated. The trend is leaning toward carbohydrate restriction, but these trends can sometimes take fifteen to twenty years until they take hold. That's when the nutrition community will sign on."

— Dr. Thomas Dayspring

The dirty little secret about all these packaged, low-fat foods? When the fat is removed, it is replaced with something that's even worse for you. And that thing is more often than not sugar. Sure, you know that sugar isn't good for you, and that it leads to all sorts of health ailments, including obesity, diabetes, Alzheimer's disease, cancer, and heart disease. But thanks to the heavy emphasis on eliminating fat from the diet from all the so-called health experts, sugar has gotten a virtual free pass for decades. In fact, it is a lot more damaging to your health than fat will ever be. By ignoring its negatives for so long, medical and nutrition experts have unintentionally made people even more susceptible to heart disease by refusing to more closely examine their vilification of dietary fat, especially saturated fat.

MOMENT OF CLARITY: "My bet is that people will become very accepting of the anti-sugar message within the next decade. They're already buying into it. But the idea that saturated fat is not deadly could take many decades to change."

– Gary Taubes

MOMENT OF CLARITY: "The reason we are scared of cholesterol and fat has to do with the fact that there are drugs to lower cholesterol and 50 percent of what we grow in America is now either corn or soy, which can easily be manufactured into low-fat products."

– Dr. Cate Shanahan

What would you say if I could show you a study that found that eating a low-fat diet produced zero benefits in relation to cardiovascular health? Well, I just happen to have one: The results of a $415 million study of 48,835 women, measuring the impact of the low-fat diet over eight years, was published in the February 7, 2006 issue of the *Journal of the American Medical Association*. The conclusion of the study authors: The low-fat diet yielded no benefits in terms of the risk of heart disease—not even a little! And yet, despite such overwhelming evidence, there was no immediate repudiation of the low-fat lie. This study, like so many others, has been virtually ignored by the nutrition and medical communities.

MOMENT OF CLARITY: "By cutting down on your carbohydrate intake and increasing your healthy fats, that alone will lower your triglyceride levels and increase your HDL cholesterol. In fact, eating more saturated fat is one of the best ways to improve your HDL, and that is probably shocking for a lot of people to find out. No one would ever think that was true. And yet it is the saturated fats that have been demonized."

– Cassie Bjork

It's time for low-fat diet proponents—doctors, nutritionists, drug companies, food conglomerates—to admit they were wrong. They have, in fact, seriously undermined the health of Americans with flawed advice and information. Maybe they were misled, like everyone else, and it's fine to admit that. But now that we know the truth, let's ask questions, set the record straight, and promote change. To refuse to do this is simply irresponsible. People deserve to hear the truth at last.

MOMENT OF CLARITY: "People have become soured on the notion that diet works because their cardiologist, primary care doctor, nutritionist, and dietitian all gave them the wrong diet. And they did the diet, gained eight pounds, increased their blood sugar levels, and their cholesterol went up a little higher. The dietitian or physician tells the patient they're not following the plan, even though they are doing it exactly. People have become very skeptical that there's any real genuine merit to diet, and that causes them to start saying silly things like 'Everything in moderation.' But while the right diet is incredibly powerful, it's not the same diet you're going to receive from your dietitian."

– Dr. William Davis

If you're wondering how we could have gotten such a vital issue wrong for so long, you're not alone. This is one of the major reasons why I wanted to write this book: to share lifesaving health information with you. Discovering that health experts are fallible, that their information is not unassailable, made me thirst for the truth so that I could take back control of my health. More and more people are doing just that every day, and if you are reading this book it means that you are either fully on board or open to joining us when you've become convinced. Either way, give yourself a big pat on the back for thinking for yourself. Far too many people are simply going through the motions of life on autopilot, expecting others to tell them how to live healthy. That's taking the easy way out and is what has led us down this deep rabbit hole of health decline.

I realize how overwhelming all this brand-new information must be for many of you. It goes against everything most of us have grown up believing is true without question. Just take it in chunks and absorb what you can. Changing everything you once believed to be rock solid truths about cholesterol, diet, and health isn't easy, especially when the message is so pervasive, as the next chapter demonstrates.

KEY CHOLESTEROL CLARITY CONCEPTS

→ **Most medical doctors have minimal education and training in nutrition.**

→ **Ancel Keys is responsible for sending us down the low-fat rabbit hole in the 1950s.**

→ **Keys's Seven Countries Study was flawed because it ignored relevant data.**

→ **The drug and food industry are still profiting from these fallacies today.**

→ **When fat is removed from a food product, it is usually replaced with sugar.**

→ **An important study found that a low-fat diet has no positive impact on heart health.**

→ **Low-fat diet recommendations for health should be called into question.**

Chapter 8

Carbs and Vegetable Oils: The Twin Villains

MOMENT OF CLARITY: "If you're living a lifestyle where you are doing everything you can to reduce inflammation and oxidative stress by reducing your consumption of carbohydrates in your diet, eating a clean, whole, unprocessed-foods Paleolithic diet and taking supplements to complement your diet, what's that going to do for your risk of developing plaque and heart disease? It's going to reduce it. In other words, those lipoprotein molecules are going to become less sensitive to harm. In this context, it almost doesn't matter what your cholesterol numbers are and you don't have to worry about it."

– Dr. Jeffry Gerber

MOMENT OF CLARITY: "I tell my clients not to stress over what their cholesterol numbers are necessarily and instead focus on eating fewer trans fats, processed refined carbohydrate-based foods, grains, and sugar, while adding in more healthy fats. That in itself is a brand-new concept to many people."

– Cassie Bjork

Let's quickly recap what we've learned so far. Cholesterol and fat in our diet are integral to our health and vitality and should not be feared. Chronic inflammation—due in part to eating sugar, blood sugar-raising carbohydrates like whole grains, and processed foods—is the true culprit in heart disease. Statin drugs may lower cholesterol levels in the blood, but they don't significantly reduce the incidence of heart attacks or heart disease, in addition to potentially also causing deleterious side effects. And, finally, the decades-old idea that a low-fat diet is some kind of nutritional panacea has been turned on its head; increasing evidence shows that, rather than being heart-healthy, such a diet raises inflammation in the blood vessels (which goes a long way toward explaining the rising rate of heart disease in America and around the world).

And, of course, there's much more to this story. In fact, these next truth bombs may be the most difficult to believe but are arguably the most important part of this paradigm shift that needs to happen in your thinking.

MOMENT OF CLARITY: "If you change from a high-carbohydrate, low-fat diet to a higher-fat, lower-carbohydrate diet, then you move into your primary energy source becoming fat. A lot of patients are coming in and are virtually 99 percent sugar burning because carbohydrates are their primary food source. That's what their body is using for fuel. When you are in that state, you just can't access fat stores—in fact, you'll be driving more fat into your fat stores. That's why it is imperative that we get people out of sugar burning, and we can now demonstrate this. Hopefully, with evidence such as this, we can further increase the strength of the message."

— Dr. Malcolm Kendrick

Carbohydrates Play a Bigger Role in Health Than You Realize

For me, carbohydrates are the dreaded "c" word, what I refer to as "carbage." It is critical to your overall health to understand the enormous impact they are having on your heart—especially refined white flour and sugar. My next book, *Keto Clarity*, deals with this issue in more depth, examining how virtually every chronic disease is tied to the overconsumption of carbohydrates and the lack of healthy fats in our diet. In the meantime, I'll focus on how carbohydrate-based foods affect you metabolically, thus increasing your risk of developing heart disease, and how they negatively and radically impact your cholesterol levels in ways that aren't necessarily reflected in your LDL and total cholesterol.

MOMENT OF CLARITY: "On high-carb diets, which most people in the general population are eating, high levels of LDL cholesterol usually indicate metabolic syndrome or hypothyroidism."

— Paul Jaminet

Consuming large amounts of carbohydrates—that is, whole and refined grains, sugars (even the natural ones from fruit, for example), and starchy foods—triggers a dangerous chain reaction in your body. The carbs you eat are composed of glucose, fructose, or a combination of the two, which then raises triglyceride levels. That, in turn, increases the number of small, dense lipoproteins that cause damage to your arteries (more on those later). How can you prevent this? It's pretty simple: by limiting your consumption of the carbohydrates that raise your triglycerides. It's a easy solution to radically improve your heart health immediately.

MOMENT OF CLARITY: "My overall philosophy is to personalize treatment as much as possible. But for most people seeking weight loss, I advocate limiting carbohydrates, particularly sugars and processed grains."

– Dr. Ronald Krauss

Consuming excessive amounts of carbohydrates is more fattening than eating saturated fats. This is a truth you won't hear from mainstream health professionals, which is why most Americans, as well as a lot of people around the world, continue to favor carbs over just about any other food. It is certainly a big reason for our epidemic of obesity, despite all the low-fat and fat-free foods lining our grocery shelves. Yet for so many decades we've blamed saturated fat for making us fat and sick. Here's the stone cold truth: You are healthiest when you consume healthy fats—as God naturally made them, in plants and animals—and dramatically reduce carbohydrates in your diet.

MOMENT OF CLARITY: "Every experiment that looked at high-fat diets as a causal factor in endothelial dysfunction used a piece of lard fed to the test subject between two slices of bread or sugary milkshakes. If you want to do a high-fat experiment, try doing it with just the fat! Every experiment has been done with a pretty high dose of carbohydrates."

– Dr. Dwight Lundell

Studies on high-fat diets have almost always been done in conjunction with a high-carb diet. We are now beginning to see that the mixture of high fat and high carbohydrate foods is a recipe for disaster, leading to an almost inevitable and rapid decline in health. Many researchers and health experts have made the mistake of targeting fat when it comes to heart disease. But what if, as evidence is beginning to show, carbohydrates are doing most, if not all, of the real damage? Unfortunately, though, carbs are not the only problem: You might be stunned to learn about another ubiquitous "health" recommendation that's directly contributing to heart disease.

Say Goodbye to Vegetable Oils

MOMENT OF CLARITY: "Most vegetable oils don't come from a vegetable at all. Instead, they come from waste products like cottonseeds or seeds specifically designed for the food industry, like canola seeds, rice bran, and things like that. These seed oils make up the vast majority of what is in food labeled as vegetable oils."

— David Gillespie

All the same health experts and organizations warning us about high cholesterol levels and saturated fat, and telling us to add "healthy" whole grains into our diet, have also been actively promoting vegetable and seed oils: corn, peanut, sesame, safflower, sunflower, and canola oils, to name a few. You also know them as the supposedly heart-healthy, omega-6, polyunsaturated fats. But make no mistake: They are among the most dangerous substances in the food supply you can put in your body.

MOMENT OF CLARITY: "Many people think I'm nuts when I flat-out say that lard and butter are better for you than canola oil."

— Cassie Bjork

Try this experiment: Take a stroll down the aisles of your local supermarket and randomly pick up any packaged food. I can guarantee that you will find, among the long list of ingredients, one of the oils I just listed. They are in everything: salad dressings, pasta sauces, doughnuts, granola bars, whole-grain breads, mayonnaise, and crackers. It seems impossible for foods to be processed without them.

MOMENT OF CLARITY: "The study looking at the Sydney Diet Heart Study data demonstrates yet again what we know—that the polyunsaturated fats, particularly those full of omega-6 fatty acids, are extremely unhealthy. And yet we have all these manufacturers creating these oils. In the UK, the British Heart Foundation recently linked up with a company that makes a synthetic margarine substance called Flora and is promoting it to consumers as the world's healthiest thing to eat. And it's full of omega-6 fats. Yet this reality doesn't seem to have an effect on them at all. It's amazing how they just carry on. But the evidence is out there and it's really strong that fats are different substances. It's saturated fat that our bodies were designed to eat. Saturated fat is the fat that your body synthesizes if you eat too much sugar. Why would the body make an unhealthy substance if saturated fat were bad for you? That's just completely bonkers!"

— Dr. Malcolm Kendrick

A meta-analysis of the statistics from the Sydney Diet Heart Study, published in the February 2013 issue of the *British Medical Journal*, dealt a severe blow to advocates of polyunsaturated fats. The stats were based on a randomized, controlled trial conducted from 1966 to 1973; the participants—458 men between the ages of thirty and fifty-nine—had all recently suffered a coronary event. The researchers sought to "evaluate the effectiveness of replacing dietary saturated fat with omega-6 linoleic acid, for the secondary prevention of coronary heart disease and death." They split the study participants up into two groups: the control group continued to eat a diet rich in saturated fats; the second group switched to a diet high in safflower oil–based foods. What exactly did this new, meta-analysis reveal?

While the group consuming the greater amounts of safflower oil predictably saw a big drop in their LDL and total cholesterol levels, these oils didn't necessarily protect them from the risk of death from heart disease. In fact, their risk was even higher than it was for those in the control group. The analysis concluded that the supposed benefits received from switching from saturated fats to omega-6 vegetable oils actually puts you at *greater* risk of having a heart attack! Yes, the fat sources heavily marketed to you and me as "heart-healthy" by the American Heart Association are actually causing the very thing they are supposed to prevent. What's wrong with this picture?

MOMENT OF CLARITY: "The oils used in cooking by most families, such as vegetable oils, are loaded with omega-6 fatty acids, and these have led to more heart disease. These fats are directly impacting your cholesterol by oxidizing it, which is leading to cardiovascular damage. If you heat up and eat a fat like soybean or canola oil, it eventually shows up in the arteries of people who have had bypass surgery. If people would just stop eating that kind of fat, they would not get heart disease."

— Dr. Fred Kummerow

MOMENT OF CLARITY: "Eat organic and avoid processed foods, vegetable oils, and sugar."

— Stephanie Seneff

We have been instructed by health experts to eat omega-6-rich vegetable and seed oils and to give up real food saturated fats like butter, coconut oil, and animal fats. Most of us have obediently complied and as a result we have seriously compromised our health. But that's not the worst part of this story. In the days following the release of this damning new science knocking the health halo off suddenly not-so-healthy vegetable oils, how did the American Heart Association respond in a press release? Did the AHA change its position on saturated fat or its heavy promotion of polyunsaturated fat? Nope.

Instead, the AHA doubled down on its position, stating that there is "a robust body of scientific studies that demonstrates a strong association between eating a diet high in saturated fat and the development of atherosclerosis, which clogs arteries and causes heart disease." The AHA spokespeople went on to repeat their recommendation to limit saturated fat consumption to no more than 7 percent of total calories consumed. And they continued to push omega-6 fats, such as sunflower, safflower, sesame, and flax seed oils. In other words, as heart disease rates continue to rise, the American Heart Association is just sticking their fingers in their ears and singing "la la la, I can't hear you" while ignoring genuine scientific data that supports the very opposite of what they are advising. I have to ask again: What is wrong with this picture?

MOMENT OF CLARITY: "Cholesterol and fat do not clog our arteries. Fatty foods are digested and packed into particles that can carry fat in our bloodstream without clogging them up, but only as long as those particles themselves are properly built. When our diets are full of corn and soy oil, or the other common, industrial vegetable oils, the lipoprotein particles do not contain enough antioxidants. Without antioxidants, lipoproteins are easily destabilized. When these fat-containing particles are destabilized, the fat they were shuttling through the bloodstream is suddenly unprotected and cannot stay suspended in the blood so it will splat onto the inner lining of the artery, just like a paintball. There, a complicated series of reactions lead to inflammation, which eventually weakens the artery wall so that it bleeds and forms a clot that we call a heart attack or a stroke. The reason LDL levels tend to go up when people follow unhealthy diets has to do with all of this. The lipoprotein is destabilized and the enzymes that are supposed to be able to get the fat inside the lipoprotein delivered to the cells are not functional. So the number of LDL particles—also known as ApoB-containing particles—suspended in the bloodstream at any one time appears to rise."

– Dr. Cate Shanahan

David Gillespie Sounds the Alarm on Vegetable Oils

One of the world-renowned health leaders attempting to blow the lid off the vegetable oil ruse hails from Brisbane, Australia. David Gillespie, another of the featured experts in this book, wrote the 2013 book *Toxic Oil*, which advocates running, not walking, away from these dangerously unhealthy seed oils as fast as you can. Gillespie's frustration over the unscrupulous marketing of omega-6 fats was apparent when I interviewed him for this book. Though truly health-enhancing omega-3 fats—those you find in wild-caught fish, local farm eggs, and grass-fed meats—are now getting more attention, they are still downplayed in comparison to omega-6 fats. "The problem with seed oils is that they are very, very high in polyunsaturated fats," Gillespie noted. "We've been told these omega-6 fats are good for us, and they are, but only in very small quantities."

Put simply, our balance is off: We're eating more omega-6 fats than the more beneficial omega-3 fats, which are typically found in flax seeds, walnuts, salmon, sardines, and grass-fed beef, among other foods. The ideal ratio of omega-6 to omega-3 fatty acids should be 1:1, with a 3:1 ratio at the very worst. In reality, most of the world has a ratio that is more like 30:1. And for that you can blame the vegetable oils used in virtually every packaged food product on grocery shelves today.

"Prior to grains being introduced into the human diet, we were probably consuming a 1:1 ratio of omega-6 and omega-3 fats," Gillespie told me. "Once grains were introduced into the food supply ten thousand years ago, that added a lot more omega-6 fats into our diet, pushing the ratio to 2:1. Nobody knows for sure, but speculation is that, from the middle of the nineteenth century until now, the ratio became more like 15:1 and, in some places, it's as high as 30:1 in favor of omega-6. The introduction of very, very cheap man-made seed oils are the reason we are now consuming more omega-6 fats than our bodies can possibly cope with."

This influx of omega-6 fats—now comprising 15 percent or more of the calories consumed by most of the world's population—is "dangerous and uncharted territory," Gillespie added. And it all leads back to inflammation, which we discussed in chapter 2.

"The pro-inflammatory mechanism in our body is driven by omega-6 fats and the tamping down of inflammation is driven by the omega-3 fats," Gillespie said. "By consuming an overload of omega-6 fats, we are pushing our system toward a proinflammatory state, which is why omega-6 consumption is now implicated in autoimmune disorders, allergic reactions, and rheumatoid arthritis."

Nobody, including Gillespie, is denying that your LDL and total cholesterol levels will drop as a result of consuming these vegetable oils. But what cost is this having on our bodies? As Gillespie pointed out, "Lowering the amount of cholesterol circulating in your body isn't a good thing if you are increasing the chances of oxidizing the cholesterol."

It's this oxidation of the LDL cholesterol that ultimately leads to a heart attack and cardiovascular disease. Oxidation in our cells is similar to metal rusting over time. In the same way, omega-6 fats degrade your cells, making them extremely fragile. Here you are thinking that you are healthy because you are using oils that reduce your cholesterol when, in reality, your body is becoming much more atherogenic—that is, more susceptible to heart disease or a heart attack. And yet few health "experts" are talking about this.

"When we consume these omega-6 fats, what we are setting ourselves up to do is to create a significant percentage of our LDL becoming oxidized," Gillespie explained. "We can now measure oxidized LDL levels, and what has become abundantly clear in the last five to ten years is that there is a very, very strong correlation between people's level of oxidized LDL and their risk of heart disease."

While the fats found in animal-based foods are often vilified for being "artery-clogging," the reality is that these natural fats do *not* become oxidized; rather, they protect against other forms of oxidation in the body. "There's a reason animal fat doesn't become oxidized—because it has to be transported in a very high-oxygen-rich environment," Gillespie said. "Just to be sure, our liver packages up those LDL particles with antioxidants—

coenzyme Q10 and vitamin E, for example—which act as little fire extinguishers on the 'fire' of oxidation."

Knowing your personal level of oxidized LDL is a "much more powerful predictor of heart disease than any other measurement we can take from our bloodstream," Gillespie added. While your cholesterol numbers can predict heart disease about 49 percent of the time; measuring for oxidized LDL predicts it 82 percent of the time. This is why Gillespie argues that we are focusing on the wrong thing—getting our LDL lower—when we should be zeroing in on the reasons why LDL is becoming oxidized.

"When you look at how heart disease develops, it just makes sense that oxidized LDL levels are a strong predictor of heart disease," he told me. "What's becoming really clear is that oxidized LDL is a very bad thing. But what's becoming more clear is that the way to make sure you've got plenty of oxidized LDL is to load up your LDL with an easily oxidized omega-6 fat."

We'll get into the various particles associated with LDL cholesterol (yes, there is more than one kind of LDL) in the next chapter, but it is the small, dense LDL particles that are particularly harmful to your overall heart health, since they can embed themselves inside your arterial wall, leading you down the path to heart disease. "Ask your doctor for a test that measures oxidized LDL," Gillespie said. "I don't know how widely available the test is, but it does exist and your doctor should be able to order it."

MOMENT OF CLARITY: "Perhaps the reason testing for oxidized LDL isn't as readily available in the United States is because there is no drug that will lower it. So there's no benefit to our healthcare system, aside from improving people's health. And the pharmaceutical companies cannot benefit because the best way to reduce oxidized LDL is by cutting sugar consumption, reducing stress, exercising, and stopping smoking."

– Dr. David Diamond

If you're having trouble measuring for oxidized LDL, there are some LDL particle blood tests you can run, which I'll explain more about in the next chapter. But before you take any tests at all, know that there is something you can do right now to improve your overall health: Replace the vegetable oils, sugars, grains, and other culprit carbohydrates in your diet with fresh, real, unprocessed foods and natural, real food-based saturated fats. Doing that will take you down the path to becoming healthier than you ever thought possible.

DOCTOR'S NOTE FROM DR. ERIC WESTMAN: One of the clips I use to teach my patients is from the documentary Fat Head. *The text goes something like this: "If you could put all of human history into one year, then we only started eating grains yesterday, and we only started consuming vegetable oil one hour ago—which is when the increase in heart disease started."*

KEY CHOLESTEROL CLARITY CONCEPTS

→ **Carbohydrates raise triglycerides, VLDL, and small LDL particles.**

→ **Carbohydrates from grains, sugar, and starch are the most fattening.**

→ **Studies looking at high-fat diets usually include loads of carbs, too.**

→ **Omega-6-rich vegetable oils, promoted as healthy, are the most damaging fats you can eat.**

→ **Vegetable oils are found in virtually every packaged food product today.**

→ **We are consuming upwards of 30:1 omega-6 to omega-3 fatty acids when the ratio should be 1:1.**

→ **Higher consumption of omega-6 fats oxidize LDL particles, which leads to heart-health issues.**

→ **Measuring oxidized LDL particles is more important than cholesterol screening.**

→ **To be healthy, switch to a real foods–based, low-carb diet with natural fats.**

Chapter 9

What's This LDL Particle Thing?

MOMENT OF CLARITY: "A total cholesterol level is useless. Cholesterol is the payload and in and of itself is not the problem. It's merely the vehicle that determines if there is a problem. When it's in HDL, it's good. When it's in large, buoyant LDL particles, it's neutral. When it's in VLDL, it's bad. And when it's in small, dense, LDL particles, it's disastrous."

– Dr. Robert Lustig

MOMENT OF CLARITY: "The least accurate way of estimating your atherogenic risk on a standard cholesterol panel would be to look at total cholesterol or LDL cholesterol."

– Dr. Thomas Dayspring

Hopefully, by this point in the book, I have made a strong case against looking almost exclusively at LDL and total cholesterol as a means of measuring heart-health risk. I might have even convinced you that the vilification of saturated fat by the health and medical communities is one of the biggest scams that has ever been perpetrated on the American public. That's a lot to digest already, but I hope you've saved room for some more. Specifically, I'd like to get into the most relevant tests for overall cardiovascular health, beginning with LDL particles. This is the part of *Cholesterol Clarity* you've been waiting for!

LDL has long been seen as the dirty word in the cholesterol conversation. But did you know there is more than one kind of LDL? What you generally see on your cholesterol test results is LDL-C, which is nothing more than a calculated number using something called the Friedewald equation. Most people don't realize that their LDL number is an *estimate* on a standard cholesterol test, not an exact number—in other words, it is calculated and not directly measured. And yet the stated goal of most doctors is to bring LDL cholesterol levels below 100. Does that make any sense at all?

MOMENT OF CLARITY: "LDL has never been looked at as an independent risk factor in any of the scientific literature. The reason for this is partly because the way of measuring it has always been so indirect. We know how to measure total cholesterol and HDL particles in the blood. For the rest of it, they do some kind of calculation [the Friedewald equation] and figure that must be your LDL cholesterol."

— Dr. Cate Shanahan

MOMENT OF CLARITY: "There's an increasing consensus that measuring particle concentrations of LDL—the whole particle, not just its cholesterol content—is a more meaningful and, in many cases, a more accurate means for assessing risk. And even more importantly, for defining goals of treatment. This whole area of particle testing has been categorized as 'emerging' technology, even though it's been emerging for three decades now."

— Dr. Ronald Krauss

Why Measuring for LDL Particles Is More Beneficial Than Estimating LDL Cholesterol

You might be wondering if there is a way to directly measure your LDL. And, lo and behold, there is! There are two major classifications of LDL particles that can be measured: Pattern A is the large, fluffy, and generally harmless kind that is described as "good" LDL (yes, there is such a thing); Pattern B is the small, dense, potentially dangerous kind that is described as "bad." Pattern B LDL can easily penetrate the arterial wall, compromising your heart health. This is what you are trying to avoid at all costs, so knowing the breakdown of your LDL particles is critical to determining overall heart health.

MOMENT OF CLARITY: "You want to have your Small LDL-P [the actual number of LDL particles contained in your blood] number as low as possible."

— Dr. Jeffry Gerber

MOMENT OF CLARITY: "If most of your LDL particles are the large, fluffy kind, then you don't have a problem and you have nothing to worry about. It's so important to know the makeup of your LDL. This is where our problem is—just looking at the LDL-C number and automatically assuming it's bad if the level is high. And yet there's such a big difference in the particle types—your LDL-C number just doesn't tell the whole story. The size of the LDL particles is so much more important than LDL-C. You want to have mostly the big, fluffy Pattern A LDL particles, and less of the small, dense, B-B type Pattern B LDL particles."

– Cassie Bjork

So how do you measure the particle number and size of your LDL? Actually, the technology for doing this has been around for a while and it has become more sophisticated over the years. Despite that, if you ask your doctor about running the particle size test, you will very likely get either a puzzled look or some comment about how it is unnecessary. Keep in mind that since cholesterol can be lowered with statin drugs, the pharmaceutical companies have been very effective in "educating" your doctor to look only at LDL and total cholesterol as the primary cardiovascular risk markers. But you can and should insist on getting one of the various tests that measure LDL particles. Your health insurance may not cover it, but I promise these tests are worth the cost.

MOMENT OF CLARITY: "Of the thousands and thousands of patients I have personally seen over the years with coronary disease, I can count the number of people who lacked a prevalence of small LDL particles on one hand. It is possible for it to happen, but it's highly unusual. The vast majority of people who have coronary disease or a risk of developing it have an excess of small LDL particles. There's only one thing that causes small LDL particles and that's carbohydrates, not dietary fat. We use a low-carb diet to eliminate the expression of small LDL, which also, by the way, reduces blood sugar levels and normalizes blood vitamin D levels."

– Dr. William Davis

The great news is that you can order many of these tests for yourself at websites like PrivateMDLabs.com, DirectLabs.com, and HealthCheckUSA. com. You don't even need a prescription from your doctor. For those of us without health insurance, myself included, that is an excellent option.

However, it is critical to find a physician who can help you interpret those results, but the information contained in this book should help. Here are three excellent resources to help you in locating a medical professional who can assist you in both running and interpreting more advanced cholesterol tests: LowCarbDoctors.blogspot.com, PaleoPhysiciansNetwork.com, and PrimalDocs.com.

To determine which cholesterol tests are right for you, let's take a look at what's available and where.

MOMENT OF CLARITY: "Many of my colleagues disagree with how these methods [of advanced cholesterol testing] should be used. They don't want to confuse practicing clinicians by bringing in anything beyond the standard cholesterol tests."

– Dr. Ronald Krauss

A Guide to Cholesterol Tests

General Lipid Panel

This is the cheapest and most common cholesterol test around, accessible in any medical facility; it requires a simple blood test in your doctor's office. This is typically referred to as a lipid (fats in the blood) panel, and it is taken after a required twelve-hour fast, usually overnight. The four primary types of lipids tested include a calculated LDL-C, HDL-C, triglycerides, and total cholesterol. Some doctors will run an extended version of the lipid panel that also measures VLDL and non-HDL cholesterol. You'll learn about these later in the book. Again, a lipid panel is typical of any annual checkup, and though you can extrapolate important information from the results, it is the bare bones basics.

Berkeley HeartLab Test (BHLInc.com)

The Berkeley Heartlab Test determines if any hereditary issues play a role in your overall heart health. It's primarily run on people with existing heart disease, who have had a heart attack, who have a family history of heart disease, or who are obese or suffering from diabetes. Various gene tests—like the ApoE genotype—are run along with LDL and HDL particles. It's a very comprehensive blood panel that uses a proprietary technology called gradient gel electrophoresis to determine the seven subclasses of LDL particles. Price and insurance coverage vary from state to state.

The VAP Test (TheVAPTest.com)

The Vertical Auto Profile Test (more commonly referred to as the VAP Test) is an advanced, comprehensive cholesterol test from Atherotech Diagnostics Lab, which does a complete analysis of your lipid panel in a fasted or nonfasted state. Direct measurements of LDL, VLDL, and HDL, as well as ApoB, triglycerides, and Lp(a), are taken along with a breakdown of the HDL. LDL density is also measured, with a breakdown of Pattern A and Pattern B, but it does not measure LDL-P. This test is usually recommended for patients with known heart-health issues, such as atherosclerosis, type 2 diabetes, high inflammation markers, and those with increased risk factors (cigarette smokers and/or people with high blood pressure, low HDL-C, a family history of heart disease, or who are middle-aged). The VAP Test costs about the same as a general lipid panel and is covered by most health insurance.

NMR Lipoprofile Test (Lipoprofile.com)

The NMR Lipoprofile from Liposcience is a state-of-the-art test for measuring your LDL particle numbers, including LDL-P and the particle size. Any physician using this test is interested in digging deeper into heart disease prevention. The standard cholesterol numbers are run, along with the LP-IR number, which assesses your susceptibility to insulin resistance. This is a highly recommended test for anyone who has been told they have high cholesterol and need to take a statin drug.

Diabetes Prevention & Management Panel (HDLabInc.com)

Health Diagnostic Laboratory offers one of the newest and most advanced cholesterol tests you can have run. You get the traditional lipid profile numbers, along with lipoprotein particles, inflammation markers, genetic markers, heart function, metabolic markers, and much more. It's a pretty cool test many of the more progressive physicians are beginning to use in their medical practice. You'll be hearing a lot more about this important cardiovascular risk test in coming years.

Ion-Mobility Spectrometry (QuestDiagnostics.com)

Ion mobility, a means for measuring lipoprotein particles from Quest Diagnostics, probably isn't on your doctor's radar just yet, but it provides the most direct, accurate, and reproducible physical measurement of both the size and concentration of various lipoproteins in the blood. It also produces much more reliable results for each of the lipoprotein subclasses of LDL, HDL, and VLDL. The precision of ion mobility is astounding and therefore highly desirable in both research and clinical settings.

Genova Diagnostics's CV Health Plus Genomics (GDX.net)

This test analyzes your blood using NMR technology, which assesses the key markers underlying cardiovascular disease, including inflammation, lipid deposits, endothelial dysfunction, and clotting factors. It provides the standard cholesterol panel and virtually all the other advanced testing markers—Lp(a), hs-CRP, ApoE genotype, and more—in one report. The insulin resistance score by lipid fractionation is unique to the Genova test.

MOMENT OF CLARITY: "Should we be checking cholesterol at all in the clinical setting? I think the answer to that is a definite yes. It is a tool that uses that standard of care in measuring cardiac risk in our patients. I use cholesterol testing to monitor the success or lack of success of dietary modification. I don't use it as a tool to recommend medication, except in those few patients who don't succeed with some type of nutritional change."

– Dr. Jeffry Gerber

Far too many people are walking around with an abundance of Small LDL-P or very high LDL-P, and they are simply ignorant that these things exist and the potentially negative ramifications they are having on their health. And that's thanks to some rather pervasive LDL-C brainwashing by virtually all of the major health organizations in the world. Now that you know the importance of LDL particle testing, you can take appropriate action: Either have the appropriate tests done yourself, or push your doctor to go beyond the basic tests that tend to focus primarily on total cholesterol and LDL-C, which don't really tell you much about your heart health risk.

In the next chapter, we'll take a look at the unwanted stepchildren of the cholesterol panel: these are the markers that get ignored by most doctors, and yet hold the key to your true risk of developing heart disease.

DOCTOR'S NOTE FROM DR. ERIC WESTMAN: Keep in mind that the whole point of measuring blood cholesterol and inflammation is to prevent or treat atherosclerosis. I recommend that my patients get their "arteries checked" for atherosclerosis periodically.

KEY CHOLESTEROL CLARITY CONCEPTS

→ There are varying sizes of LDL cholesterol.

→ Traditional LDL cholesterol is merely a calculated number on your test results.

→ Pattern A LDL cholesterol is large, fluffy, and generally harmless.

→ Pattern B LDL is small, dense, and potentially dangerous.

→ You should have one of several particle tests conducted to assess your risk.

Chapter 10

Forgotten and Ignored: Triglycerides and HDL

MOMENT OF CLARITY: "There isn't a drug that lowers triglyceride levels well, which is why mainstream medical doctors don't pay much attention to them. But triglycerides respond very strongly to dietary changes. If you reduce your carbohydrate intake, you tend to have ideal triglyceride levels, in the 50 to 60 range. Additionally, the triglyceride-to-HDL ratio is a good indicator of how well your diet is dialed in. If the ratio is high, you might benefit from eating more saturated fats and fewer carbs."

— Paul Jaminet

I remember having my cholesterol tested with a standard lipid panel in early 2005, after losing 180 pounds the year before. My regular family doctor was out of the office on the day I went in to get the results and his analysis of my numbers. After looking at my test results, the fresh-out-of-school physician's assistant filling in for him gazed up at me with a disturbing look of consternation. My total cholesterol was (to him) a shockingly high 225, and my LDL reading was a ghastly 130. He was adamant that I needed to be on a high-dose statin drug pronto.

When I inquired about the stellar ratio between my HDL cholesterol (72) and my triglycerides (43), he admitted that those numbers were certainly in the good range, but quickly dismissed them as irrelevant to heart health. Keep in mind that I had just come off statin medications in 2004, and I had brought my weight down from 410 pounds to 230 pounds and was therefore getting healthier. He acknowledged that my triple-digit weight loss was impressive, but still wrote me a prescription for 40 mg of the cholesterol-lowering statin drug Lipitor.

MOMENT OF CLARITY: "People have got to understand that the mantra of 'LDL cholesterol is bad' and 'HDL cholesterol is good' is wrong. Cholesterol does so many important things; you should be glad if you have a lot of cholesterol going to your cells. The fact that your LDL might be up isn't a bad thing. The notion that it is has absolutely no basis in scientific fact. It's just used to scare people and to sell statins."

– Dr. Donald Miller

MOMENT OF CLARITY: "Triglycerides are as tied to heart disease as LDL. There are two kinds of LDL: the large, buoyant variety that is not associated with heart disease, and the small, dense variety, which is definitely associated with heart disease. The best way to determine which LDL you predominantly have is by looking at your triglycerides level. High LDL and high triglycerides mean you have a preponderance of Small LDL-P, insulin resistance, and metabolic syndrome. That is what I am looking for when I run a cholesterol panel."

– Dr. Robert Lustig

MOMENT OF CLARITY: "The triglyceride–to–HDL-C ratio should not be used in African-Americans. They just don't have high triglycerides, even though they have severe insulin resistance. Why? Because they have different types of lipase, the enzymes that catabolize triglyceride expression. And this has been well written about. In fact, African-American cardiologist Dr. Keith Ferdinand has been hammering this message. So the triglyceride–to–HDL-C ratio message is great, but don't go there if you're an African-American. Their insulin resistance is better characterized by glucose abnormalities, obesity, and high blood pressure, not high triglycerides and low HDL cholesterol. The sad part is that almost nobody, not even healthcare providers, realize this."

– Dr. Thomas Dayspring

I had to wonder why HDL or triglycerides are even measured in the first place if they aren't as important as LDL. Don't they mean anything? Why would you just discard them as unimportant when they are right where they need to be? But this physician's assistant—with all of his training fresh in his mind—simply dismissed them in favor of focusing on my "bad" LDL numbers. There's one simple explanation: those he could "fix" with a statin prescription.

You'd think that in a supposedly modern age, doctors would realize that every patient is unique and there is no one blanket treatment for everyone. I told the physician's assistant point blank that I would not go back on a statin drug because the side effects I experienced were far too serious for me to ignore. I asked him for a natural way to get my LDL down if that was supposed to be such a bad thing. To my surprise, he did offer an option—albeit without very much enthusiasm. He gave me a pamphlet from the Orlando-based Florida Lipid Institute called "Drug-Free Cholesterol Lowering Plan," a program developed in 2003 by Dr. Paul Ziajka.

The pamphlet recommended a low-fat "lifestyle change" and advised replacing eggs, cheese, butter, and red meat with tofu, baked chicken, low-fat cheese, 1 percent milk, and margarine. Yuck! Additionally, the pamphlet included a three-component plan for getting cholesterol down: plant stanols, soy, and soluble fiber. Plant stanols, such as Benecol and Take-Control, help prevent the absorption of cholesterol; soy supposedly lowers cholesterol numbers (and even that is now being questioned); and soluble fiber helps lower cholesterol in the GI tract. If you followed this plan, Dr. Ziajka promised a 45 percent decrease in LDL and a 35 percent decrease in total cholesterol.

The pamphlet ended with his sentence, which made me chuckle:

Following our plan and a low-cholesterol, low-fat lifestyle can cut your cholesterol level in half! Just remember, these are changes you are going to make the rest of your life.

A low cholesterol, low-fat lifestyle for the rest of my life? I don't think so! I've done the low-fat diet and it just plain didn't work for me. My low-carb lifestyle is doing just fine to keep me healthy, thank you very much. To adopt the pamphlet's plan would have meant abandoning the lifestyle changes that helped me lose triple-digit weight and get my health back, and that wasn't about to happen.

Before I left my doctor's office I asked again about testing for other kinds of LDL. The physician's assistant filling in for my doctor dismissed the idea again (and in all honesty, my doctor would have said the same thing), saying the additional tests were simply too unreliable and cost-prohibitive to bother with. His discouragement of looking further into the numbers was both shocking and depressing. How many other patients interested in challenging the conventional wisdom—treating their high cholesterol with a statin medication and a low-fat diet—were being subjected to this song and dance from the very people we have entrusted with our health?

MOMENT OF CLARITY: "Triglycerides and HDL are good biomarkers for measuring someone's risk for developing heart disease. My extreme combination of high triglycerides and low HDL put me at a fifteen times greater risk of developing heart disease. I don't think it's prudent to ignore these biomarkers, but rather to educate ourselves about what they mean to our health. That's why I decided to become enlightened about why I was gaining weight and what I could do about my abnormal lipid levels."

— Dr. David Diamond

DOCTOR'S NOTE FROM DR. ERIC WESTMAN: The more I read articles, perform research, and follow patients in my clinic, the less concerned I become about the traditional way of looking at their blood cholesterol levels. I don't even worry about blood cholesterol for the vast majority of people who have basically normal levels. Medical doctors were taught—and then we taught our patients—that cholesterol in the blood is a bad thing; that LDL cholesterol is lousy or lethal and that HDL cholesterol is healthy. And, because the pharmaceutical companies have only been able to create medications that lower LDL, we have not heard much about HDL. American medicine has a way of quashing minority opinions. Maybe in our rush to create guidelines or in the competitive nature of pharmaceutical companies we have forgotten how to do true science. The reality is that there have always been a group of scientists and clinicians who never believed in this flawed interpretation of cholesterol—men like Dr. Gerald Reaven, most famous for identifying metabolic syndrome, and Dr. Robert C. Atkins, who popularized the low-carb, high-fat diet. Instead, they emphasized the importance of lowering triglycerides and raising HDL cholesterol. They didn't know the reasons for this back when they were making these proclamations, but they knew that addressing these blood components could be helpful to the patients dealing with obesity and chronic disease. Now, with greater scientific precision, we know just why triglycerides and HDL are a much better pair of numbers to look at than LDL-C and total cholesterol.

MOMENT OF CLARITY: "Relying on total cholesterol alone is just bad medicine. It's 1960s thinking, and this was effectively the stone age of lipidology. The science has evolved dramatically since then."

— Gary Taubes

MOMENT OF CLARITY: "I think the focus was so overly intense on looking at LDL and total cholesterol that triglycerides escaped scrutiny for a while. Without getting into details, high triglycerides trigger the production of the small, dense lipoprotein particles that are now thought to be integral to the oxidative and inflammatory processes that cause arteriosclerosis."

— Mark Sisson

DOCTOR'S NOTE FROM DR. ERIC WESTMAN: By now you have learned that having mostly Small LDL-P is bad, since that ultimately leads to atherosclerosis, and that these small, dense LDL particles greatly increase when triglycerides are simultaneously high and HDL cholesterol is low. If you want to look at something on your standard lipid panel to determine your cardiovascular risk, simply figure out the ratio of triglycerides divided by HDL cholesterol to assess the triglyceride-to-HDL ratio. This number goes hand in hand with determining whether or not you have a prevalence of small LDL particles. When the triglyceride-to-HDL ratio is high, there are more small LDL particles. Conversely, when the triglyceride-to-HDL ratio is low, there aren't many small LDL particles at all, meaning that you are at a reduced risk of heart disease.

MOMENT OF CLARITY: "I always look at the triglycerides first. And if they are under 100 and closer to 50, then I'm happy with that. More than anything, I look at the triglyceride-to-HDL ratio with an optimal goal to be as close to 1 or lower."

— Cassie Bjork

DOCTOR'S NOTE FROM DR. ERIC WESTMAN: An interpreter is often needed to explain what all this means to the patient. It's not unlike speaking a foreign language. But even people in the medical profession, who are taught to focus only on LDL, don't understand the triglyceride-to-HDL ratio concept. That's why we need to enlighten doctors so they can help their patients, as I am doing in my own clinical practice. Doctors like myself need to be agents of change at the grassroots level, educating as many fellow physicians and patients as we possibly can.

Knowing Your Triglyceride-to-HDL Ratio Is Critical to Assessing Heart-Health Risk

MOMENT OF CLARITY: "If you don't have access to measuring your Small LDL-P, the next best markers to look at are your triglycerides and HDL. You should bring these into line, and not according to the usual guidelines that you may see on your cholesterol panel. Having triglycerides of 150 is complete nonsense. Aiming for less than 50 is more like it. And with HDL, I'm not happy until we're seeing about 50 or higher. Ideally, I prefer this number to be 70 to 80 or higher. If you have low triglycerides and high HDL, then it is possible you may have small LDL, but probably not a lot."

– Dr. William Davis

Have you ever paid much attention to what your triglycerides or HDL numbers are on your cholesterol panel? Did you even know what they were prior to reading this book? For most people, the answer is no. But as my co-author Dr. Westman notes above, these are the two critical cholesterol panel numbers that you should be paying a lot more attention to. Simply looking at LDL-C or total cholesterol won't help to predict cardiovascular risk as effectively as learning that, for example, your HDL is over 50 and your triglycerides are under 100. Ideally you want a 1:1 triglyceride-to-HDL ratio. Do you want to take a wild guess at what you can do to bring this ratio into perfect balance? Cut your carbs and increase your fat. This is a recording.

MOMENT OF CLARITY: "The biggest marker of poor cholesterol health is elevated blood levels of triglycerides, which is one of the most important biomarkers for determining your overall metabolic health. There is a strong inverse relationship between triglycerides and HDL cholesterol."

— Dr. Dominic D'Agostino

Triglycerides are a type of fat in the blood linked to heart disease and stroke, and yet you probably have never heard of them. The medical establishment has lavished all their attention on LDL cholesterol. Personal experience made Dr. David Diamond, one of the featured experts quoted in this book, dig a little deeper; his extremely high triglyceride level prior to 2006 could not be ignored. What he came to understand was that, yes, carbohydrates are the primary driver of triglyceride production.

MOMENT OF CLARITY: "The most common cause of high triglycerides is eating too many carbs."

— Paul Jaminet

MOMENT OF CLARITY: "High triglycerides are an indicator of impaired energy metabolism in the cells because they are less able to use sugar for fuel. Therefore, the body has to keep these fats elevated in the blood to be available as food for the cells that can't get the sugar. The reason they become unable to manage sugar is because they don't have enough sulfate. Sulfate is needed in order to store sugar, so you end up with high blood sugar levels and high triglycerides."

— Stephanie Seneff

Dr. David Diamond's Triglycerides Challenge

The general recommendation for triglyceride levels is 150 or less. In the late 1990s, Dr. David Diamond's numbers began to rise; by 2006 his triglycerides were at a whopping 800! We now know how shocking that is, but back then no one was putting much stock in triglycerides, so he simply ignored the numbers. His total cholesterol was a relatively low 220, and he felt fine. But something more obvious was changing. "Over the years I had gained weight—about twenty-five pounds since graduating college—and as I became noticeably overweight I grew concerned about my health," Diamond told me. "Weight gain may be one of the most important biomarkers because it's an obvious sign that something is wrong."

In 2006, his doctor finally got concerned. In addition to Diamond's high triglyceride levels, his HDL cholesterol was very low. The cause turned out to be a genetic predisposition to elevated triglycerides, and his doctor told him that nothing but medication could lower the numbers. But Diamond wanted to find a more natural solution. He began to educate himself and hit upon a stark realization that changed his thinking forever. "There's one very simple way to elevate triglycerides and that is eating simple carbohydrates," Dr. Diamond states. "It's not the dietary fat that makes high triglycerides, it's the sugar!"

Just by cutting down on carbohydrates, Dr. Diamond saw his triglycerides drop from 800 to below 150. He never took any medication. "Interestingly," he said, "my HDL cholesterol level doubled from an abysmally low 25 to a very healthy level of 50. So my numbers are great now, and it's all thanks to the changes I made to my diet."

HDL Cholesterol Is Closely Tied to Your Triglycerides

HDL is absolutely tied to your carbohydrate consumption as well as your fat intake. Consuming fewer carbs and more healthy saturated fats like butter, full-fat animal foods, and eggs will bring your HDL levels up quite nicely. If the positive health effects routinely seen on a low-carb, high-fat diet were accomplished instead through drugs, the medical profession would be calling it the most astonishing breakthrough in the medical treatment of cholesterol and cardiovascular health treatment ever. But since it's just a dietary change and there is no real money to be made in promoting that, the reaction from health experts is the equivalent of a collective yawn. Improving health and curing disease naturally should be more important than profit, of course, but that's not how the world works. It's unfortunate, but money clouds the judgment and motives of otherwise good people.

MOMENT OF CLARITY: "Sure, saturated fats can increase your cholesterol, but mostly by increasing HDL cholesterol and making more of the big, fluffy LDL particles and less of the small, dense bad ones."

— Cassie Bjork

Fortunately, no one is stopping you from taking charge of your own health, and paying more attention to your triglyceride and HDL numbers is a giant step in that direction. Coming up in the next chapter, our experts explain some of the other things worth watching that you may not have heard before. It's chock full of practical information, so get ready to soak it up!

KEY CHOLESTEROL CLARITY CONCEPTS

→ **Medical doctors tend to ignore triglycerides and HDL cholesterol.**

→ **Enlightened clinicians no longer worry about traditional cholesterol results.**

→ **True science should be about questioning conventional wisdom, and that's not happening.**

→ **High triglycerides and low HDL cholesterol make for elevated levels of bad LDL.**

→ **Measuring the ratio of triglycerides to HDL is critical to assessing heart health.**

→ **Carbohydrate consumption drives triglycerides higher.**

→ **Cut the carbs and your triglycerides will fall, without taking drugs.**

→ **Eat more saturated fat to raise your HDL cholesterol levels.**

→ **If a low-carb, high-fat diet were a drug, it would be heralded as a scientific breakthrough.**

Chapter 11

The Experts Weigh In on Key Heart-Health Markers

MOMENT OF CLARITY: "Debunking the cholesterol myths is a message that needs to get out because the misinformation is a bad thing being done to people."

– Dr. Donald Miller

We've spent most of the book so far explaining why, when it comes to heart health, LDL and total cholesterol numbers are overrated, while triglycerides, HDL, and LDL particle numbers are underrated. We've also stressed that inflammation and oxidation are the true causes of heart disease. And we've debunked the low-fat-diet myth, exposing the evils of our carbohydrate-rich and omega-6 oil laden diets. Throughout the book, my experts have weighed in with periodic "Moment of Clarity" quotes that hammer home what we are sharing with you. If there is a heart to *Cholesterol Clarity*, it is the wisdom gleaned from these doctors, researchers, nutritionists, and enlightened health gurus. So why not give them a chapter all their own?

What follows is a rapid-fire potpourri of intelligence from my esteemed experts. This is arguably the most informative chapter in this book once you grasp what is being shared in these pages more fully. Some of the concepts, ideas, and language will be brand new to you. Once again, don't worry if you don't understand everything they say; all will be explained in due course. Now prepare to be astounded!

MOMENT OF CLARITY: "We know now that oxidation and inflammation are the true drivers of heart disease. More and more physicians are beginning to understand this. But the most powerful 'medicine' in this case has proven to be food; what you do and do not eat can have the greatest impact when it comes to altering blood lipids and reducing risk of heart disease. This represents a personal power that people haven't experienced in medicine before, a realization that they are not necessarily doomed to be victims of unlucky family genes, and that they can control their health by understanding the power of food and exercise."

— Mark Sisson

MOMENT OF CLARITY: "If you look at the advanced lipid tests—LDL-P, ApoB, and the size and density of the LDL—then heart disease becomes a carbohydrate problem. As long as you're focusing on LDL cholesterol as the culprit, then you can blame saturated fat."

— Gary Taubes

MOMENT OF CLARITY: "Lowering the triglycerides number is most important to me because that's the number that really increases with the consumption of processed carbohydrates, sugars, and trans fats. If you can get that number close to 50 or lower, you will see improvements overall. I also like checking the hemoglobin A1c (HgA1c) number, which measures the consistency of your blood sugar levels over time; ideally, that number should be under 5.0. And, of course, I pay attention to the C-reactive protein (CRP) marker, which is a telltale sign of systemic inflammation; those levels should be under 1.0. If you have an increased CRP but you don't have any infection going on, that may mean that there is blood vessel inflammation. It wouldn't be shocking to me if someone with high CRP levels also had cholesterol levels that are high; that's because your body is sending cholesterol to repair a problem. If I see a client with a CRP level below 1, then I'm not concerned about what the cholesterol level is. It's really hard to communicate this message to people because their doctor has only warned them about their cholesterol levels. Once I gain people's trust by showing them something that works, they begin to trust me more than their doctor. When we're talking about inflammation, I like to look at what's causing it. If the client's CRP levels are high, I want to look for the root cause of the inflammation—smoking, excessive alcohol consumption, consuming trans fats and processed carbs, high blood sugar levels, chemical exposure, high blood pressure, and stress can all contribute to this. Everything on this list veers from common medical wisdom, which immediately blames inflammation on a high-fat diet."

— Cassie Bjork

MOMENT OF CLARITY: "It's very clear that the things you should be most concerned about with your lipids are your HDL and your VLDL, otherwise known as your triglycerides level. When your HDL level is low and your VLDL level is high, this means your metabolic system is out of whack. It is a very important sign of underlying issues, like insulin resistance and metabolic syndrome, which are the things you should really be worried about bringing under control. These are important signs that your health is in danger."

— Dr. Malcolm Kendrick

MOMENT OF CLARITY: "Elevated homocysteine levels are a risk factor in heart disease. It's actually a much stronger risk factor number than LDL cholesterol. And there's no drug to improve homocysteine without making matters worse. Homocysteine (a protein amino acid) is very interesting because it is a precursor to sulfate. In order for homocysteine to become sulfate, it has to have oxidation damage. Homocysteine induces inflammation in the blood vessels leading to the heart and gets trapped in the artery wall along with plaque to produce sulfate. Sulfate deficiency is the key problem behind all modern diseases. Everything comes back to this. Sulfate deficiency is caused by a combination of three things: a severe reduction in the availability of sulfur in food because of food processing, exposure to environmental toxins, and lack of sun exposure. Our bodies require sulfate to detoxify our bodies from the chemicals we are exposed to from plastics, pesticides, and aluminum. For example, glyphosate is the active ingredient in Roundup, which is widely used as a weed killer. Glyphosate actually disrupts sulfate transport and sulfate synthesis. Sunscreens often contain aluminum, which disrupts sulfate synthesis in the skin. Sunlight catalyzes sulfate synthesis in the skin. So if you're avoiding the sun and putting on sunscreen, you're preventing your skin from producing cholesterol sulfate. The skin is the major supplier of cholesterol sulfate to all the tissues, but thanks to various lifestyle choices, our skin is not able to do its job."

— Stephanie Seneff

MOMENT OF CLARITY: "Reducing any inflammation in the body and eliminating stress are the most important and effective ways to lower cholesterol. In order to do that, you need to get enough sleep, exercise, and, most critically, eat correctly—and by that I mean switching to a low-carbohydrate diet. In all my years of practicing medicine, it's the one thing that does the most in helping to bring cholesterol levels down."

— Dr. Fred Pescatore

MOMENT OF CLARITY: "There are many arguments for the view that cardiovascular diseases are caused by infections. More than fifty different bacteria and viruses have been identified in atherosclerotic arteries, but none in normal arteries. The symptoms of an acute heart attack are the same as those of infections: slight fever, raised sedimentation rate, and leukocytosis. Atherosclerotic tissue is often inflamed, and today many researchers believe that atherosclerosis is caused by the inflammation. We disagree; the inflammation is the result of an infection. Inflammation is necessary—it is our body's way of combating infection—and, consequently, all trials with anti-inflammatory drugs have resulted in more heart attacks."

— Dr. Uffe Ravnskov

MOMENT OF CLARITY: "The plain fact is that measuring cholesterol levels cannot tell you much about someone's risk of heart disease. And even if it did, what would I do with the information that my cholesterol is elevated? Personally, I'm unlikely to take statins because the chance of my benefiting from them is very small and the risk of unwanted side effects is much higher. If I wanted to preserve the health of my heart, I might make a concerted effort to eat a natural, unprocessed diet, be active, optimize my vitamin D levels, avoid smoking, etc. But I already do all those things. In other words, knowing my cholesterol score would not change anything, so there's no point in knowing it. That's why, when I am asked what my cholesterol level is, I say: 'I don't know, and I don't need to know as it won't make a difference in how I manage my health.'"

— Dr. John Briffa

MOMENT OF CLARITY: "In the general population, there are dozens of studies—done with hundreds of thousands of people—that, when pooled together, suggest that the total–to–HDL cholesterol ratio is the strongest independent blood lipid–based predictor of cardiovascular disease and mortality."

— Dr. Chris Masterjohn

MOMENT OF CLARITY: "HDL is very good and you want your HDL levels to be high, but not by artificially raising them with a medication. You can do it naturally through cutting your carbohydrates, increasing fat consumption, and exercise."

— Dr. David Diamond

MOMENT OF CLARITY: "You can get the micronutrients you need by eating animals 'nails to tail.' Getting good micronutrients and improving gut health is vital to healthy lipid profiles."

– Paul Jaminet

MOMENT OF CLARITY: "I look for several things. I like to see a good, solid HDL number that is at least 10 points higher than what most labs consider 'normal' values. Triglycerides should be under 150; I don't believe as strictly that triglycerides must be below your HDL number as long as they are below 150. And finally, I check the fasting glucose and hemoglobin A1c."

– Dr. Cate Shanahan

MOMENT OF CLARITY: "If your triglyceride–to–HDL-C ratio, a free calculation, comes back as abnormal, it's money well spent to go get an ApoB or LDL-P done. ApoB is readily available in any lab in the country. Diabetics, pre-diabetics, and insulin-resistant patients especially have residual risk and should have this test done routinely. Is there anything predictive in a traditional cholesterol panel where there's a little bit less discordance with ApoB and LDL-P? It comes down to non-HDL cholesterol calculated by simply taking total cholesterol minus HDL cholesterol. Total cholesterol is the sum of cholesterol that is in your ApoB particles, which is not in your HDL particles. Theoretically, the cholesterol that is in the HDL is not supposed to hurt you because HDLs do not deliver sterols into the arterial wall, so I'm really interested in your ApoB cholesterol. This non-HDL number provides you with your ApoB cholesterol number. That's why non-HDL cholesterol would be a better biomarker than is LDL-C, and it's a free calculation that average people should be looking at instead of their LDL-C number."

– Dr. Thomas Dayspring

MOMENT OF CLARITY: "If you're still looking at LDL as the 'bad' cholesterol, then you're about thirty years out of date; we found out that LDL had different forms about twenty years ago. It could be that really bad cholesterol—the small, dense LDL particles—is the main problem for most obese and diabetic patients. So how do we predict small, dense LDL? The easiest way is if your triglycerides are elevated and your HDL is low. Elevated triglycerides and low HDL signals the onset of obesity and metabolic syndrome, a prediabetic state that's already been defined."

– Dr. Ken Sikaris

MOMENT OF CLARITY: "There are a lot of people who are fearful of making these kind of changes, but you can reduce your cardio-metabolic risk by decreasing your dose of statins gradually while simultaneously trying the nutritional changes that are effective for improving your overall health. Look at your triglycerides, HDL, or maybe even your LDL particles or ApoB number, to assess how you are doing. This is a way for people to dip their toe into this new way of thinking—reducing inflammation as opposed to lowering cholesterol."

– Dr. Philip Blair

MOMENT OF CLARITY: "Insulin resistance is important because it is the root cause of atherosclerosis. A random blood sugar level above 120, lots of small particles or Pattern B LDL cholesterol, remnant lipoproteins, elevated CRP levels, low GlycoMark, and A1c around 5.0–5.3 are the things that make me want to work up a patient more earnestly. You don't really need to do fancy advanced lipid testing; triglycerides, HDL, and non-HDL numbers are available on every standard lipid panel."

– Dr. Rocky Patel

MOMENT OF CLARITY: "Look for hidden genetic causes for heart disease. It's a growing list, but the two most common genetic causes are Lipoprotein(a)—what I consider the most powerful cause for heart disease that nobody gives a damn about—and a genetic tendency to overexpress the small LDL."

– Dr. William Davis

MOMENT OF CLARITY: "The up-regulation of proinflammatory pathways associated with high blood sugar and insulin is going to be more detrimental to your cardiovascular health than elevated cholesterol."

– Dr. Dominic D'Agostino

MOMENT OF CLARITY: "The standard cholesterol test—as commonly given in the United States—is the last thing I would look at in assessing cardiovascular risk. The first thing I'd want to know is the triglycerides-to-HDL ratio. When it comes to the current state of your health, this ratio is one of the most telling numbers on your entire blood panel, and a great substitute for insulin resistance and for the expensive cholesterol particle testing. The particle test is the only cholesterol test with any real value because it tells you the number and size of your LDL and HDL particles. If you cannot get the particle test done, the triglycerides-to-HDL ratio is a good indicator as well. A high number here almost always signifies a large number of small, dense LDL Pattern B particles, which is not good. But the LDL-C number alone is meaningless."

— Dr. Jonny Bowden

MOMENT OF CLARITY: "Dietary cholesterol is not the problem in heart disease. We've shown that in a study I published in the January 1979 issue of the *American Journal of Clinical Nutrition*. You can check for oxidized LDL with a urine test."

— Dr. Fred Kummerow

MOMENT OF CLARITY: "The JUPITER study proved that the very best marker of cardiovascular risk is C-reactive protein, which detects inflammation. The study focused on a population of people having cholesterol levels of 130 or below and elevated CRP; half the group took a statin drug and the other half got a placebo. Lowering inflammation is key in the prevention of heart disease."

— Dr. Duane Graveline

MOMENT OF CLARITY: "I always talk about getting the biggest bang for your buck in clinical medicine, and for me the bottom line is basic tests that reveal levels of inflammation and oxidative stress. So I look for markers of insulin resistance. Checking for adrenal function and thyroid function is important, too."

— Dr. Jeffry Gerber

MOMENT OF CLARITY: "The general population, rather than worrying about cholesterol, should start paying attention to their postprandial [after eating] sugars. To me, the key to health is controlling your blood glucose levels following a meal to less than 140. Think about diabetic patients. They have chronic, intermittent hyperglycemia and their endothelial cells—in a set of particular vulnerable areas— are diseased and die. They go blind, they lose their kidney function, they have their legs amputated, they die of premature heart disease, and they have neuropathy. It happens because all these endothelial cells can't resist the glucose barrage the way other parts of the body can. Rather than trying to modify all the metabolic pathways with medications, why not try eliminating sugar from the diet? We're seeing more and more information in the medical literature associating insulin levels with diseases, but nobody is asking how we are getting high insulin levels."

— Dr. Dwight Lundell

MOMENT OF CLARITY: "Going from the top, total cholesterol is the least reliable lipid marker. LDL cholesterol is also not so good. Non-HDL cholesterol is better. LDL particle concentration is even better. You could also include ApoB concentration because it's very similar."

— Dr. Ronald Krauss

MOMENT OF CLARITY: "Get rid of the toxins in your life that lead to inflammation: chemicals in your food, air, and water; household cleaning products; cosmetics and personal hygiene products; pharmaceuticals and nutraceuticals; pathogens; genetically modified organisms; oxidized cholesterol; polyunsaturated oil; and heavy metals."

— Dr. Ron Ehrlich

MOMENT OF CLARITY: "If I narrowed it down to just a few tests, I'd look at someone's waist circumference, uric acid, fasting insulin, and lipid profile as my general metabolic screening."

— Dr. Robert Lustig

MOMENT OF CLARITY: "People will often ask me, 'If cholesterol doesn't cause heart disease, what does?' Basically I tell them it's four things: vitamin deficiencies, particularly A, D, E, and K2, as well as the B vitamins 6, 9, and 12; a low-fat diet, which usually means low saturated fat and high-carbohydrate consumption; polyunsaturated fats and stress. Of the three factors, the one that plays a particularly damning role in heart disease is the lack of vitamin K2."

— Dr. Donald Miller

DOCTOR'S NOTE FROM DR. ERIC WESTMAN: For metabolic risk assessment, first check the serum glucose, then the serum triglyceride and HDL, then, if you can, the LDL size—are they small or large? I realize this is a book on cholesterol, but just focusing on cholesterol and not glucose as well would be incomplete.

As you can see, all these leading and enlightened health experts have come to the same conclusion: Looking at LDL and total cholesterol as the primary markers of the state of your heart health is simply ludicrous and lazy. There are more important things to pay attention to. In the next chapter, we'll take a look at why most doctors cling to such archaic, out-of-date theories about cholesterol.

KEY CHOLESTEROL CLARITY CONCEPTS

→ **Food is the most powerful "medicine."**

→ **Triglycerides, A1c, and CRP reveal more about heart health than total cholesterol.**

→ **Homocysteine levels need to be brought under control for optimal health.**

→ **Infections can lead to an increase in inflammation, resulting in heart disease.**

→ **High HDL cholesterol is a good thing.**

→ **Lipoprotein(a) and genetic tendencies for small LDL are often overlooked.**

→ **Testing for oxidized LDL in the urine is something everyone should be doing.**

→ **Check insulin, and blood sugars to assess overall metabolic health.**

→ **Measuring waist circumference and uric acid levels are excellent indicators of overall health.**

Chapter 12

Why Are So Many Doctors Clueless about Cholesterol?

MOMENT OF CLARITY: "When we learned that cholesterol was there in the arteries, treating it became the standard of care. And the drug companies very quickly swooped in to influence the science in this field. They didn't do it by bribing doctors ... it was much more sophisticated than that. I can remember a time when they got me to give a talk, they made me an opinion maker, they funded my research, they got their people on FDA panels, and they were part of creating the National Cholesterol Education Program. So as standards of care came in, if you came into my office with elevated cholesterol and I did not treat you with a statin drug, then my treatment was considered below the standard of care. So physicians today basically have no choice but to recommend treatment with statin medications for anyone with elevated cholesterol."

– Dr. Dwight Lundell

Becoming a doctor is a hard road; it takes years of education and a big financial investment. But the rewards can be great, and what could be nobler than devoting your life to healing people from disease? Let me say it again: I have the greatest respect for the nurses, doctors, naturopaths, dietitians, chiropractors, and other healthcare professionals who make this sacrificial commitment to the betterment of others. They deserve our utmost respect and gratitude.

That said, I am troubled by how little most traditionally trained medical doctors are taught about the nutritional component of health. Sadly, much of what they learn is based on the theories pushed by Ancel Keys (whom we discussed earlier) and George McGovern; he was the politician responsible for getting the government involved in making standardized national dietary recommendations decades ago. But what about all the twenty-first-century research that disputes Keys's rather shifty science? Apart from the experts quoted in this book, the mainstream medical community seems determined to stick with outdated and potentially dangerous ideas. That's truly baffling to me. Isn't part of the Hippocratic oath to "first do no harm"?

MOMENT OF CLARITY: "We've been giving people the wrong advice for the past fifty to sixty years. And instead of admitting that we have gotten it all wrong on obesity and chronic disease, we now think we should push the message even harder. It's like zealots: They can't change their minds because they are incapable of doing so."

– Dr. Malcolm Kendrick

Some of the most frustrated e-mails I receive from my blog readers concern their doctors' responses to their cholesterol results. It saddens me that, in light of all we are learning about the irrelevance of LDL and total cholesterol, doctors are still encouraging misguided fears and pushing unnecessary drugs predicated on these two numbers alone. As I said in chapter 5, statin therapy works for the small percentage of people who refuse to adapt to a healthier lifestyle. But for the most part, these drugs are overprescribed to patients who don't need them. Let's take a look at a few of these e-mails.

MOMENT OF CLARITY: "There's a sort of convenience issue to provide numbers that doctors will remember to treat to."

– Dr. Ken Sikaris

▸ My doctor wants to put me on a statin drug to lower my 225 total cholesterol and 147 LDL cholesterol. I obviously said no because my HDL is 70 and my triglycerides are 41.

▸ I was diagnosed with type 1 diabetes at the age of fifty-three. I now follow a low-carb, Paleo-style diet. I recently had my cholesterol numbers run and my doctor prescribed a low-dose, 10 mg statin—but I am *not* taking it! My total cholesterol is 234 with LDL-C at 139. My HDL is 85 and my triglycerides, which run high in my family, are 148. I don't want my darn doctor prescribing medications that will end up giving me more problems. By the way, I weigh ninety-five pounds so there isn't much I could cut in the way of eating other than carbs.

► My cholesterol saga began in 2006 when I was diagnosed with type 2 diabetes. My doctor noted that my total cholesterol was high at 199 with an LDL cholesterol of 165. My HDL was low at just 28 and my triglycerides were borderline high at 154. My fasting blood sugar levels were 258 and my doctor wanted to get that down immediately. A couple of months later, he wrote me a prescription for Lipitor since he wanted my LDL cholesterol below 100. I was willing to take the statin but my wife warned me about the side effects. In researching these, I came across the work of Dr. Duane Graveline and other cholesterol skeptics, which motivated me not to fill the Lipitor prescription. That is when I discovered a low-carb diet for diabetes and gave it a try. When I finally returned to the doctor, expecting a confrontation over my not taking the cholesterol-lowering drug he had prescribed, imagine my surprise when my LDL had dropped to 101—without ever taking a single medication. Needless to say, there was no more talk about taking a statin drug. My LDL has stayed around 100, my HDL cholesterol rose, and my triglycerides came down below 100. I still can't believe my doctor never told me about the power of a low-carb, high-fat diet to improve my cholesterol numbers!

► I recently changed doctors and my new doctor noticed in my chart that I had a total cholesterol of 246, LDL 157, HDL 70, and triglycerides 97. She asked me if my other doctor had discussed putting me on a statin medication and I explained to her that my previous doctor said I did not need to because my HDL was really good, which was protecting my heart, and that all the relevant ratios on my cholesterol panel were really good. She just ignored me and had the office call in a prescription for a statin. I called the office back and was told that my high LDL cholesterol alone warrants medication. I informed them that I refused to go on a statin due to my excellent ratios.

► My cholesterol used to be stellar when I was a carbohydrate-addicted vegetarian. Sure my triglycerides were high and I was obese, but dang, I had a total cholesterol below 130! Then I switched over to eating low-carb, started eating meat, and dropped seventy pounds. My HDL went up, but so did my LDL cholesterol. The nurse-practitioner at my doctor's office freaked out when my total cholesterol came back at 252. I explained to her that I wasn't concerned, but she was having none of it.

- I was on Crestor for about a year and took myself off it shortly after going on a low-carb diet. I just had my annual physical and got my blood-work numbers back with a total cholesterol of 210, up from the 127 level I saw while taking the statin drug. Not surprisingly, the doctor wants me to go back on Crestor again. UGH!

- My total cholesterol of 185 causes my primary care physician to shout *statins* from the rooftops whenever she sees me.

MOMENT OF CLARITY: "There are multiple factors at work that explain why most physicians and medical professionals only tend to look at LDL-C and total cholesterol in assessing the cardiovascular risks in a patient. The top reason is the lack of self-education by doctors; they're just not willing to open their eyes to some of these issues. And unfortunately, a lot of it has to do with the system itself. We have a healthcare system that pushes quantity over quality. Unfortunately, we only get paid based on the number of patients we see. And we're in a system, especially in primary care, where we don't get paid very well compared to our specialist colleagues. Yet the preventive aspect of what we could do as primary care physicians could save billions of dollars. It's a system that has driven us into seeing a high volume of patients, and spending very little time with them; averaging only three to seven minutes of face-to-face time. So you're in and out without a lot of time to do lifestyle coaching or making therapeutic changes. Also, you have to pay your increasing overhead costs while insurance company reimbursements are going down."

– Dr. Rocky Patel

Take Action
Just Because Your Doctor Is Shortsighted Doesn't Mean You Have to Be!

As we have stated often in this book, the vast majority of doctors seem to zoom in on just two numbers on your cholesterol panel: total and LDL cholesterol. Ideally, they say, total cholesterol should be below 200 and LDL cholesterol should be under 100. Who came up with these magic numbers? Ask most physicians that question and you'll probably get an answer like, "Well, that's the standard we've always used." But why? As you've already

learned, there is no measurable improvement to heart health when cholesterol numbers are reduced to those seemingly arbitrary levels.

MOMENT OF CLARITY: "The problem is the cholesterol laboratory is telling doctors what to think about the numbers they are testing. Seeing is believing. You forget any new information you may have heard at medical conferences be-cause you keep seeing it in black and white in every single patient you do a test on. That's a huge, huge part of all this. Why aren't the lab values changing to fit with the latest science? It's because the laboratory directors are not going to rock the boat and jeopardize their careers. They don't want doctors calling them up and saying, 'What the heck? This is not what I've heard.' They're going to stick with the status quo. That is probably 95 percent of the reason why we are still mired in this old thinking regarding cholesterol."

– Dr. Cate Shanahan

You also now know how most primary care doctors treat a "high cholesterol" problem: They tell you to lower your fat intake, exercise more, and
take a statin drug like Lipitor or Crestor, which can cause some rather disturbing side effects to your health that are far worse than any supposed
high cholesterol danger.

MOMENT OF CLARITY: "Many doctors simply look at your chart or at the computer and totally ignore you as the patient. But they need to look at you. From a doctor's standpoint, the first thing I want to see is how my patients walk into the room, how they are behaving, whether they are alert, what their color looks like, whether they have any swelling. But we've stopped doing that in the medical profes-sion. This seems to be a lost art and can't possibly be done in a ten-minute office visit every three months. Patients are mere data points and doctors have no idea what's really going on with their health. The primary mission of doctors should be to make people feel better. How can they do that if they're not even looking or thinking about that when a patient comes to see them? Too many physicians are trying to do a mechanical thing rather than considering the patient's overall welfare. And actu-ally, patients can choose whether they want to go through any given therapy or not."

– Dr. Philip Blair

So considering how the healthcare system is stacked against patients,
I'm doubly impressed when my readers tell me that they are standing up to

pressure from their doctors. Whether they are refusing to fill a prescription for statins or shifting their focus to nutritional therapies, I commend them for taking control of their own health. Just because your doctor's knowledge of nutrition is limited doesn't mean yours needs to be.

MOMENT OF CLARITY: "One potential problem here is that when doctors and scientists learn something and have it quite well established in the psyche, we generally find it very difficult to let go of these thoughts. I think we don't change our stance on things as often as we should, even when faced with overwhelming evidence. Even when the facts seem to change, we fail to change with them. Some of this has to do with our rejection of facts that do not fit with preconceived ideas, but also I don't think we should ignore the fact that the pharmaceutical and food industries have the ability to befriend and groom 'key opinion leaders' who can be paraded in front of clinicians, researchers, and the media. They can earn good money and derive significant kudos, too, and this may be difficult for some people to turn their backs on."

— Dr. John Briffa

But how do you, with no medical training, convince doctors, with all their training and years of experience, that they are wrong about cholesterol? My own doctor listens to what I have to say, but his ideas are still very much deeply rooted in conventional wisdom based on his education and personal experience with his patients over the years. It is intimidating, even for me, to question authority; I, too, worry about insulting my doctor or making him angry. This is natural. But keep in mind that good doctors are in the business of making their patients healthier; they get just as frustrated by poor results as you do. So if, for example, your health improved because you opted to try a low-carb diet, you might inspire your doctor to think outside the cholesterol box he's stuck in.

One medical doctor I interviewed on my podcast a few years back put it this way: The patient is always the boss, and the doctor is the employee; you have hired him to consult you about your health. But you are the final arbiter when it comes to your health.

MOMENT OF CLARITY: "Sadly, we can't always rely on our doctors for straight talk and intelligent, insightful answers. As a result, it's becoming incumbent upon patients to educate themselves, engage with others online who are providing information about nutrition and health, and go into the doctor's office as empowered patients. Doctors do help every once in a while, but they usually just hand patients some silly prescription."

– Dr. William Davis

MOMENT "I think average people are making a big mistake going to the doctor to get their cholesterol checked. That simply puts them on the **OF CLARITY:** road to being given a poison for a disease that isn't a disease! People have to understand that what seems like the norm is the completely wrong thing to do for your health. The most unfortunate part is that the doctors don't know any better"

– Dr. Donald Miller

The system of treating high cholesterol has got to change somehow, whether it's from the top down, with doctors moving away from overprescribing statin drugs, or from the bottom up, when people like you and me improve our heart-health risk factors through natural dietary and lifestyle changes. And seeing is believing: Most of the physicians I interviewed for this book, as well as my coauthor Dr. Westman, became convinced of the value of dietary changes after witnessing results in their own patients. Be the example to your doctor!

MOMENT "Doctors have this simplistic idea that if they can just make the numbers look good, then everything is hunky dory. But they make **OF CLARITY:** the numbers look good by feeding you some toxin that's going to disrupt some biochemical pathway. That's a really stupid thing to do! But that's exactly what they've done with statin drugs. Statins are a toxin and it disrupts the ability of the liver to make cholesterol ... That's absolutely the worst thing you can do to your body. Cholesterol is so vitally important to all the tissues."

– Stephanie Seneff

Let your doctor go through all the standard treatment protocols he needs to do to remain in medical compliance, even if that includes his writing you a prescription for a statin. But that doesn't mean you are required to fill it! This keeps your doctor out of trouble for not treating your high cholesterol properly, thus protecting him legally if something happens to your heart health. Then, try a low-carb diet filled with fresh, unprocessed foods and healthy fats. I'll bet you will see the numbers we've been discussing throughout this book improve naturally. A growing number of physicians are willing to be educated about this; they would like to move away from statins because of the harmful effects they are seeing on the health and quality of life of their patients. Empower them by proving the benefits of placing lifestyle over artificial change with a pill.

MOMENT OF CLARITY: "It takes a lot of education to overcome the brainwashing that has been taking place for years regarding cholesterol. I spend a lot of time in my sessions with clients talking about blood sugar levels and hormones like glucagon, insulin, leptin, and ghrelin. We talk about metabolism and the mainstream dieting advice that tells us a calorie is a calorie. What clicks with people is if they've tried this advice before and it didn't work; then it makes sense that there has to be a better way. When you get into the underlying biochemistry and how the body works, people realize it's a lot more complex than they have been led to believe."

– Cassie Bjork

One of my blog readers shared an extraordinary story with me about an encounter she had with her family doctor after losing over a hundred pounds eating a low-carb, high-carb diet. The doctor was thrilled with her weight loss but was concerned with her elevated cholesterol numbers. Rather than settling for being a slave to a prescription drug for the next umpteen years, she decided to do her own research. She found some invaluable information on my blog, and, while most patients simply give in to the demands of the man in the white coat, she grabbed back control of her health. She is living proof that sometimes the patient can teach the physician. Here is her e-mail:

Hi Jimmy,

I hope you don't mind me contacting you, but I want to share some things with you.

My doctor is thrilled with my 103-pound weight loss (thanks to low-carb). But I just had my blood work done a couple of weeks ago and he called me with my results. My cholesterol is even higher and he said since my mom had a heart attack way too early in life, he is concerned about me.

He said I either need to start taking a statin drug now or, if I want to try on my own, through diet and exercise, he will give me another six to eight weeks to check me again. He tells me if it's the same or higher, he wants me to go on the prescription.

I have to say that I have not been exercising, and lost most of my weight in the last one-and-a-half years. I have been thinking I should start exercising, but just haven't done so on a regular routine. But I have been dancing around the house while doing housework and making myself move more! My puppy dogs think I am trying to play with them and they get all excited. Hee hee! I have PCOS [polycystic ovary syndrome], which leads to diverticulitis and some pretty bad attacks. Needless to say, I stay away from foods that bother me.

The doctor said I needed to get more fiber, but I can't have beans or raw veggies on my low-carb lifestyle. I've been eating creamy peanut butter on a low-carb tortilla or just by the spoonful. I am totally allergic to any and all cheeses, even sour cream and cream cheese. There are also a lot of foods with smells that bother me and I just can't eat them. So my food choices are very slim, but I certainly haven't been starving while being on low-carb.

My doctor recommended that I eat more chicken than red meat and that I should consume lots of fruits and veggies. All my life when I eat fruit I don't feel good because of the sugar. I am not diabetic and get tested often, but they always say there are no signs of it. It's because of the PCOS, apparently, and my body is insulin-resistant and can't properly process carbs and sugar. I had two small pieces of cantaloupe over the weekend and my tummy was not happy with me.

After talking to my doctor, it scared me, naturally, and I started searching online and so did my hubby. He found an old blog post of yours from 2007 where you interviewed Dr. William Davis, the cardiologist who advises his patients to live a low-carb lifestyle and is in the Milwaukee, Wisconsin area. So am I! I started reading other links and posts from your blog where you and others were saying their doctors were giving them high cholesterol reports and wanting to put them on statin medications. Some had heart scans done and all was fine, meaning they didn't have to take any prescriptions after all. So that got me to thinking and I called Dr. Davis's office to find out the name of the imaging place close to me that does heart scans. I called and made an appointment and went and had a heart scan done to see for myself where I stood.

The lady who did the scan showed me the images on the computer afterwards and showed me what to look for and she said she couldn't see any plaque buildup. Yay! I got my written report in the mail a few days later and, sure enough, I got a big fat 0 (yes a zero!) on my heart scan! The normal reading for a sixty-year-old woman like me is at least 25 percent. They sent my doctor a copy of the report and I made an appointment with him to go over these test results.

When my doctor walked into the room, he was all smiles and said my heart scan report was the best it could possibly be. He said it is absolutely terrific to have a zero calcium deposit score at sixty years old. He said he didn't feel I needed to take any cholesterol medicines after all and he was actually pleased that I took the initiative and got the heart scan done on my own. He asked me how I found out about Dr. Davis and the heart scan, so I told him all that I had learned from your blog and the links you provide.

He asked me what made me want to have the heart scan done, so I told him I wasn't excited about taking any medicine if I didn't need it. That's when I started looking online and found your blog post. He was pleased that I was taking such an active role in my own health. I felt empowered as a patient that day and it was good to make my doctor feel proud of me for taking control of my own health. I sure feel better and he does, too.

Who knows, maybe this has opened his eyes a little and he now realizes that not everyone who has a high cholesterol report needs to take a statin drug. Maybe he will advise other patients to have a heart scan done before putting them on those medicines. He didn't say that, but I suppose it's possible that he might change how he treats his patients.

Thanks so much for all that you do for everyone. You and Christine and all of the others who work so hard in the low-carb community are wonderful. I enjoy reading the posts, but I tend to not to comment a lot or I'd be on the computer all day long and wouldn't get anything else done! Thank you for being you and for helping everyone and for being such a wonderful inspiration!

Wow! That's a perfect example of how an educated and empowered patient can change the course of her health, and potentially the health of others. When you refuse to believe that medication is the *only* option for changing your health, then you will do what this reader did: learn more about alternative tests and have them done, whether your doctor wants you to or not. I often ask my podcast guests why patients are so willing to consume a risky medication without first exhausting every possible natural option. Most of them say that it has to do with growing up believing that you can trust your doctor, and the physician's oath to "do no harm." Why would they prescribe a drug if it were not safe and effective? But that paradigm is now beginning to shift. What would happen if we all followed the lead of the inspiring woman above?

MOMENT OF CLARITY: "Isn't it funny that people are turning to people like Jimmy Moore for answers to their health problems rather than their own doctors because the doctors have no damn idea what's going on? Most of them haven't cracked open a textbook since 1985 and have maybe done some light reading of medical journals over the last thirty years. The new trend is the deeply engaged and empowered patient who seeks health information because it affects him personally. And so patients are turning to each other for information. People like Jimmy Moore know a hell of a lot more about these things than 99 percent of primary care physicians and my cardiologist colleagues."

— Dr. William Davis

DOCTOR'S NOTE FROM DR. ERIC WESTMAN: I hardly ever use a prescription pad since I changed from a typical internal medicine practice to one that addresses nutrition. I use my knowledge about medicine now to help my patients get off their medications safely. I sought out my own training by conducting clinical research and by attending meetings of the American Society of Bariatric Physicians.

And here's the kicker to the high cholesterol myth: By lowering it, as most doctors insist, you may actually be doing *more* damage to your health—heart and otherwise. That's right, new evidence shows that having too low cholesterol is worse than high cholesterol. If you or someone you know thinks that a total cholesterol level under 150 is a good thing, then you won't want to miss the next chapter.

KEY CHOLESTEROL CLARITY CONCEPTS

→ **Medical professionals should be respected for their commitment to patients.**

→ **There's a disconnect between chronic disease and the role nutrition plays.**

→ **Doctors use scare tactics to get their patients on statin drugs.**

→ **Take back control of your own health rather than relying solely on doctors.**

→ **Be the example of powerful lifestyle change.**

→ **Work with the protocols your doctor must go through to be compliant, then do what's right for you.**

Chapter 13

What Do You Mean My Cholesterol Is Too Low?

MOMENT OF CLARITY: "No one is researching the problems associated with low total cholesterol levels, around 140 or 130. So there are not a lot of papers on it. But we do know that people who have low cholesterol tend to have a higher risk of cancer and a higher propensity for violent suicidal tendencies."

– Dr. Chris Masterjohn

For most of this book, we've been discussing the commonly held belief that having high cholesterol levels can put you at greater risk of having a heart attack or developing heart disease. But have you ever stopped to think about the ramifications of having too low cholesterol levels? Well, why would you? Not many doctors are talking about this, but evidence is mounting that low cholesterol might be a far more serious health concern than anyone, your doctor included, even realizes.

MOMENT OF CLARITY: "Skinny people, fat people, marathon runners all get heart attacks. For the runner, it's probably because his cholesterol is too low. Having too low cholesterol is actually much worse than having too high cholesterol. Cholesterol is part of every cell in the body and plays a role in keeping those cells healthy. So to think that you need to reduce cholesterol and cut down on the amount of it that you eat is just absurd."

– Dr. Fred Pescatore

A friend of mine from church told me about the excellent cholesterol numbers he got back from his doctor. His total cholesterol had come in at 112, with an HDL of 32. My friend was a bit concerned about his HDL, since the lab range showed that this number should be over 40. I explained to him that while his HDL could indeed be better, his low total cholesterol is potentially an even bigger concern. He told me that his blood sugar and blood pressure were both fine, but that his grandfather had died of a heart attack at the age of sixty-two. Interestingly, he also had a low level of total cholesterol. Could they be connected?

The Dark Side of Low Cholesterol

One of our experts in this book is the brilliant young nutritional scientist Dr. Chris Masterjohn. He has researched the issue of low cholesterol through the study of a condition known as Smith-Lemli-Opitz syndrome. People with this genetic disorder are unable to make enough cholesterol and thus have very low levels. Here's how Dr. Masterjohn describes their physical condition: "They tend to have cranial facial deformities and deformities in various body parts, such as fingers and toes, as well as the heart and other internal organs. They also tend to have severe digestive disorders, pretty severe visual impairments, a significant increase in the risk of infection and terrible neurological development associated with autism, mental retardation, failure to thrive, and aggressive and self-injurious behavior."

For people with Smith-Lemli-Opitz syndrome, the treatment is a diet heavy in cream and egg yolks. Unfortunately, the syndrome also causes poor digestive issues, so the diet must be taken with an FDA-approved supplement that raises cholesterol (yes, raises it!). This diet and supplement, taken in tandem, essentially reverses Smith-Lemli-Opitz syndrome symptoms. And that proves, according to Dr. Masterjohn, the importance of having adequate levels of cholesterol in your body: "We can see from this that cholesterol plays an incredibly important role in the brain; neurological development; mental health; proper development of the face, the limbs, and the organs; resistance to infection; proper digestion; and basically everything associated with life."

MOMENT OF CLARITY: "Isn't it convenient that all the discussion about cholesterol by the professionals tends to ignore studies that show that half of people with 'normal' levels of LDL cholesterol are having heart attacks? The response to this from the medical industry was to lower the targets for cholesterol even more!"

– Dr. Philip Blair

Many people having heart attacks have levels of cholesterol that are commonly believed to be healthy. And that sort of misguided thinking has led to far too many tragic deaths. The untimely demise of *Meet the Press* anchor Tim Russert in 2008 is one famous example of this.

MOMENT OF CLARITY: "I think it's reasonable to ask if we should be putting people through routine cholesterol screening at all. The preferred marker right now is LDL cholesterol. But levels of this are not a very reliable marker for heart disease, and most people who have heart attacks have normal or low levels of LDL cholesterol."

– Dr. John Briffa

Tim Russert's "Perfect" Cholesterol Numbers

Tim Russert had his first heart attack as he was preparing for the show he anchored, *Meet the Press*, and it instantly killed him. He was just fifty-eight. Ironically, Russert had been doing everything that his doctors advised him to do to prevent a heart attack: He was taking a statin drug, another medication to lower his blood pressure, and faithfully riding an exercise bike everyday. Here's the most shocking part of this story: his total cholesterol was just 105! And yet his very first heart attack was fatal.

MOMENT OF CLARITY: "When cholesterol levels fall below 200 mg/dl, your immune function is suppressed and there may be negative health effects. As your cholesterol levels drop, your risk of dying from cancer and infectious disease increases dramatically. There are a wide variety of health problems that become more common as total cholesterol drops below 200 mg/dL. Nearly every healthy person around the world has total cholesterol over 200 mg/dl. There are a few people with genetic mutations that lead to low cholesterol. But in general, having low cholesterol suggests you are either eating a lipid (fat) deficient diet, such as a vegetarian or vegan diet, or you have some kind of health problem like an infection or hyperthyroidism that is lowering your LDL."

– Paul Jaminet

According to Russert's doctor, he didn't have type 2 diabetes, nor did he have any blood sugar issues. His A1c was in the normal range and his cholesterol was considered very healthy. For all intents and purposes—

and according to the modern medical convention of looking at health on paper—he was the epitome of perfect health. We now know, posthumously, that Russert had coronary artery disease and was being treated for it, but his doctor apparently didn't know how severe it was. But even if he had known, the likely course of treatment would have been a higher statin dose, a diet even lower in fat, and maybe some more exercise. In all likelihood, none of those supposedly prudent strategies would have prevented this heart attack and unfortunate death at such an early age from taking place.

MOMENT OF CLARITY: "For women, the higher their cholesterol is, the longer their life; there's a direct relationship between the two. Your cholesterol cannot be too high if you are a woman, but it can certainly be too low. We actually have a cholesterol deficiency problem, not a cholesterol excess problem. It's hard for people to believe this because they've become so convinced that excess cholesterol is bad. They can't even reframe their mind to think that way."

— Stephanie Seneff

Most doctors would look at Russert's total cholesterol number and see nothing but health. They would extol the virtues of the statin drugs that artificially put his cholesterol numbers within the so-called "acceptable" range. But what good did it do him in the end? People were perplexed and confused by his death, but no one seemed terribly angry about it. I find that response to this incredibly strange. People should have been outraged—but they weren't. Russert's health was not only made worse by modern medicine, but his death was almost entirely preventable!

MOMENT OF CLARITY: "When we were a non–insulin resistant country, all we had to deal with were genetic lipid disorders. We had high cholesterol levels that correlated nicely with ApoB or LDL-P. But when people started eating too many carbs, our insulin resistance genes suddenly began expressing themselves. That led us down a path where triglyceride molecules started to invade the LDLs and HDLs, thereby displacing the cholesterol molecules. As a result, cholesterol was looking great, but then you have a sudden death like Tim Russert's. His high triglycerides resulted in low total cholesterol and LDL-C and very high ApoB and LDL-P, paradoxically raising cardiovascular risk by dropping LDL-C. Unfortunately, he also had a lot of atherosclerotic plaque that ruptured, which led to a thrombus, coronary artery occlusion, and myocardial infarction. If clinicians working with such patients would pay a little more attention to non-HDL cholesterol, they would not be so reas-

suring to those patients that their great LDL cholesterol levels are somehow protecting them against a fatal heart attack. Tim Russert was like so many insulin-resistant
or type 2 diabetic patients: a dead man walking."

— Dr. Thomas Dayspring

The Negative Effects of Low Cholesterol on Your Heart and Brain

A study published in the January 22, 2007 issue of the medical journal
Laboratory Investigation revealed a scary fact about low cholesterol. Lead
researcher Dr. Yin-Xiong Li, assistant professor of pediatrics and cell biology at the Duke University Medical Center in Durham, North Carolina, conducted an independently funded basic-science study on zebra fish embryos
and cholesterol supplementation to prevent fetal alcohol defects. The study
revealed the critical role that cholesterol plays in tissue and organ repair.
Specifically, it helps produce stem cells. If cholesterol is too low, blood vessels become stiffer and are more likely to break. Based on this finding, Dr.
Li concluded that statin drugs are dangerous because of their cholesterol-
lowering effects. Furthermore, if levels of cholesterol are too low, there is an
increased risk of death. The right amounts and the right kinds of cholesterol in the body are so important, he went on to say, that levels should not be
reduced to an arbitrary number, like the current recommendation of 200.

MOMENT OF CLARITY: "The brain contains only 2 percent of the body mass and 25 percent of the body's cholesterol. This suggests that the brain might
actually need cholesterol. Cholesterol is incredibly important in the synapse to
transmit the message from one neuron to another. You do not want to have cholesterol deficiency in your brain. This can directly lead to Alzheimer's disease."

— Stephanie Seneff

In other words, cholesterol helps our bodies to heal. Without proper
amounts of it, we can't repair inflammation or battle infection. It also has a
profound impact on brain function. Among other things, it impacts serotonin, which regulates our moods. Indeed, adverse mental side effects are
connected with low cholesterol levels, and these can be quite traumatic,
with people reporting frequent bouts of intense unhappiness and a higher

likelihood of suicidal behavior. This is why antidepression medications tend to increase cholesterol levels. Now think about the potentially serious consequences resulting from a doctor pushing patients—particularly elderly patients—to lower their LDL below 100 or even 70. Scary, right?

MOMENT OF CLARITY: "If you lower the number of lipoproteins in your body by taking a statin drug, then you are preventing an essential healing substance from doing its job. It's an advantage to have high levels of both LDL and HDL cholesterol. People with low cholesterol have a higher risk of infection, and cancer is also associated with low cholesterol—probably because at least 20 percent of cancers are caused by microorganisms. More than twenty studies have shown that old people with high cholesterol live the longest; I've never seen a study showing the opposite. Some cardiologists scoff at my assertions about high cholesterol and respond by saying that those with high cholesterol have already died. But they forget that more than 90 percent of those who die from a heart attack or a stroke have passed the age of sixty-five."

– Dr. Uffe Ravnskov

Cholesterol Indoctrination Has Led Us to Believe Lower Is Better

Here's my pithy response to people who challenge me on the subject of cholesterol: *Prove that it is unhealthy!* They can't. If anyone questions you on this, ask this one simple question: "Can you provide any scientific proof of an undeniable connection between elevated cholesterol levels and an increased risk of developing heart disease?" The fact is there isn't any. Rather, study after study shows that it is more dangerous to have cholesterol levels that are too *low*.

MOMENT OF CLARITY: "The mortality curve is essentially flat for people with total cholesterol levels of 160–240 mg/dL. In fact, there's some evidence that shows that the higher the level is, the longer you will live."

– Dr. Malcolm Kendrick

Decades of monolithic thinking, regarding the dangers of high cholesterol and the supposed benefits of low-fat diets, makes it incredibly hard to convince people that eating saturated fat is actually good for you. I'll admit that this was the hardest concept for me to wrap my head around. But it only takes seeing successful results to become a believer—and then you want to tell the whole world about it!

MOMENT OF CLARITY: "When you look at the studies examining cholesterol, there's very little evidence that lowering cholesterol does you any good. There's a lot of evidence that shows that a lower cholesterol level is actually bad for you, but it is ignored. More than twenty studies show that people with low cholesterol don't live as long as those with high cholesterol. They just deteriorate quicker."

– Dr. Donald Miller

In the next chapter, we'll examine nine of the most prominent reasons why you may have high cholesterol. Keep in mind that high cholesterol is not itself a disease. But it can certainly be a sign that something else in your body may be out of whack.

KEY CHOLESTEROL CLARITY CONCEPTS

→ **Having low cholesterol is arguably more dangerous than high cholesterol.**

→ **People with genetically low cholesterol experience horrific physical side effects.**

→ **Adding cholesterol back into the body essentially reverses these symptoms.**

→ **Tim Russert died of a heart attack at the age of fifty-eight with a total cholesterol of just 105.**

→ **Most doctors would have looked at Russert's numbers and considered him healthy.**

→ **There's a greater risk of death from a heart attack or stroke if cholesterol is too low than if it is too high.**

→ **Low cholesterol can lead to anxiety, depression, even suicidal thoughts.**

Chapter 14

Nine Reasons Why Cholesterol Levels Can Go Up

MOMENT OF CLARITY: "Being scared of high LDL or total cholesterol is an unfounded fear. It seems everything our grandparents and great-grandparents did was right! Having a lot of butter, meat, cheese, and eggs in your diet is the way they stayed healthy. The obesity rate a hundred years ago was just 1 in 150. Now that we've cut that stuff out of our diets and replaced it with carbohydrates, polyunsaturated fatty acids, and trans fats, two-thirds of the population is overweight or obese. It's really an incredible epidemic."

– Dr. Donald Miller

MOMENT OF CLARITY: "People tend to split into camps on the issues of cholesterol. One side sees total cholesterol as the cause of heart disease and the other side says total cholesterol doesn't matter. My take on it is more nuanced because cholesterol in the blood is not the cause of heart disease. So whenever we see that total cholesterol or LDL cholesterol is high, we have to approach it in a more pragmatic way. It's not necessarily time to panic in fear of having heart disease, but also we should not approach it as if it doesn't matter, either. I think your cholesterol test results can be an important metabolic marker that can provide clues to look further into the clinical picture to see if something might be wrong."

– Dr. Chris Masterjohn

MOMENT OF CLARITY: "I tell people not to fret as much about that cholesterol number on a piece of paper and instead look at what they're eating and how they're feeling."

– Cassie Bjork

Let's say you are doing everything right with your diet and in your lifestyle but your cholesterol numbers are still high. This would naturally make you wonder what that means and if it's a legitimate concern you should try to do something about. So in the interest of crystal clear clarity, here are nine of the most common reasons why your cholesterol levels may soar higher than what is considered normal:

1. Hypothyroidism

Overweight people often talk about having a "messed-up thyroid." The thyroid is responsible for so many bodily functions, including cholesterol levels in the blood, so it's an easy scapegoat. When thyroid function is low (aka hypothyroidism), cholesterol tends to increase. What's going on with the thyroid when this happens? The thyroid hormone known as T3 tells the LDL receptors in your body to get rid of the excess LDL in the blood by pushing it into the cells, where it is used for a variety of purposes. Unfortunately, when your T3 levels are low, this process slows down, leaving LDL cholesterol floating aimlessly through your bloodstream.

I spoke with Paul Jaminet, author of *The Perfect Health Diet* and one of this book's experts, about this to gain further insight into what is happening. He advises getting a full thyroid panel for anyone with high cholesterol. But he also warns that the standard ranges on most lab reports are not very reliable. Here are two excellent books on thyroid health: Datis Kharrazian's *Why Do I Still Have Thyroid Symptoms When My Lab Tests Are Normal?* (ThyroidBook.com) and Janie Bowthorpe's *Stop the Thyroid Madness: A Patient Revolution against Decades of Inferior Thyroid Treatment* (StopTheThyroidMadness.com). I've interviewed both of these authors on *The Livin' La Vida Low-Carb Show* podcast in episodes 382 and 383.

Sometimes hypothyroidism doesn't manifest itself until you make changes in your diet. So if your cholesterol suddenly skyrockets after beginning a low-carb, high-fat or Paleo diet, get your full thyroid panel checked. In addition, make sure you are getting adequate amounts of iodine (found primarily in seaweed and kelp).

MOMENT OF CLARITY: "When cholesterol levels are elevated, we take a look at the thyroid and tend to normalize thyroid by supplementing with iodine. Thyroid dysfunction is a very common cause of hypercholesterolemia."

— Dr. William Davis

MOMENT OF CLARITY: "Anybody with any lipoprotein abnormality needs to get their thyroid checked. Clearly that can be treated if that's an issue."

— Dr. Thomas Dayspring

2. Eating Too Many Carbohydrates or Too Much Sugar

MOMENT OF CLARITY: "To me, an elevated cholesterol level is important for one reason and one reason only: It reflects that you are eating too much carbohydrate in your diet. We know that dietary carbohydrate has a huge impact on LDL; total cholesterol; HDL; small, dense LDL; fluffy, big LDL; etc. What is it that will lower LDL cholesterol? Cut your carbs."

— Dr. Dwight Lundell

Hopefully, by this point in the book you realize the powerful role food plays in connection with cholesterol. When it comes to the consumption of carbohydrates, sugars, and starches, the news is not good for your LDL. It's not so much that your LDL-C, a calculated number, increases, but that the size of the LDL particles decrease and become denser, which is what is most damaging to your heart health. This is why particle-size testing (which we discussed in chapter 9) is so critically important. When you eat an abundance of carbohydrates, your Small LDL-P, LDL-C, VLDL, and triglycerides all increase dramatically like clockwork.

MOMENT OF CLARITY: "If you have excess sugar in the blood, then the sugar attaches and attacks the LDL and causes something called glycation damage. Proteins in the blood get glycated by excess sugar; this is strongly related to diabetes. When you have diabetes, you have high sugar in the blood, and that sugar attacks the proteins in the blood. One of the things that it attacks is the LDL. Think of a keyhole gummed up with ice, preventing you from getting into your car. Your body can have the same problem. The LDL is gummed up with sugar and it becomes inefficient in delivering its goods to the tissues, so you need more of it to function properly. When LDL gets gummed up with sugar, it can't get recycled by the liver. So you get these small, dense LDL particles that are basically crud. They're garbage that can't be gotten rid of. And those are really, really bad. It gets stuck in this form, which your body can't use. That's why these macrophages come into the plaque and scavenge—to basically sweep this LDL into the cell, clean it up, and send it back out again in HDL. The macrophages are performing a very heroic activity in taking the small, dense LDL out of circulation. The LDL particle provides a service of delivering cholesterol and fats to the tissues. This leaves it as a small, dense LDL particle that then gets transported back to the liver to become refurbished and cleaned up. That process gets stuck because of the sugar."

— Stephanie Seneff

Too many people believe that blood cholesterol is raised when we eat too much fat or cholesterol. It sounds logical, but, in fact, what increases fat in your blood is eating carbohydrates. Triglycerides are the fat most closely associated with your carbohydrate intake. Consuming too many carbs in your diet will raise your triglyceride levels. Reduce carbs and your triglycerides drop like a rock. There's a definite and undeniable correlation. So here's an easy solution to reducing your cholesterol levels: Lay off the carbs! The best way to know if you are controlling your carbohydrate intake well enough is to see your triglycerides dip below 100.

DOCTOR'S NOTE FROM DR. ERIC WESTMAN: One way to remember that eating carbohydrate leads to an increase in blood and liver fat is to compare it to the French delicacy foie gras, a "fatty liver," created by force-feeding carbohydrate (corn or, in Roman times, figs) to a goose. The same thing happens in humans.

MOMENT OF CLARITY: "Habitual carbohydrate consumption prevents optimal oxidation of fatty acids for fuel. If you feed a high-carb and high-fat diet to an animal and then you draw blood and spin it down to collect the plasma, it looks like a milky-colored fat suspension. The reason for this is that the fatty acids in the diet are being spared by glucose and these triglycerides remain elevated in the blood. Your blood fats will therefore be elevated in a high-carbohydrate diet. That's what confused researchers a few decades ago, when they started seeing an improvement in triglycerides for people on a high-fat diet. What happened was the high-fat diet was controlling appetite, causing the body to oxidize these fatty acids for fuel. So this made the blood levels of triglycerides go lower. The elevated blood levels of the most proinflammatory fats are the ones brought on by a high-carb diet."

– Dr. Dominic D'Agostino

3. Consuming a Low-Carb, High-Fat Diet

MOMENT OF CLARITY: "We do see some elevations in total cholesterol, especially the LDL, in some of our patients on a low-carb diet. Most doctors have put too much emphasis on the LDL cholesterol number being the 'bad' cholesterol, and it's very difficult to change that thinking. What we tell our patients is that we're going to find out what the problem is and help them feel better. Once they start feeling better, they see the evidence that they are in fact improving. They feel life is worth living again, no matter what their cholesterol test results or their doctors have to say."

– Dr. Philip Blair

Whoa, whoa, whoa, wait just a minute, Jimmy! Didn't you just say that if I cut my carbohydrate intake my cholesterol levels would drop? Yep, I sure did. So now you're telling me that a low-carb, high-fat diet might be the reason why cholesterol levels go up?

I wouldn't blame you if you were thoroughly confused at this point. But here's the deal: When you start replacing the sugar, starch, and whole grains in your diet with healthy, real foods like red meat, eggs, and cheese, your cholesterol panel is going to change—for the better! In fact, you can count on your HDL cholesterol going up to healthy levels (well over 50), your triglycerides plummeting (definitely under 100), and your LDL particles becoming primarily the larger and fluffier kind—the Pattern A type that you want. These are all signs that you are eating well; the numbers don't lie.

But there is a segment of the population that has a mysterious reaction to low-carb, high-fat diets: Their LDL-C, LDL-P, ApoB, and total cholesterol numbers spike dramatically. The reason for now is unknown.

MOMENT OF CLARITY: "LDL-P does tend to increase significantly in a small segment of those people who eat a low-carbohydrate, high-fat, high-saturated fat diet. The question is how small is this segment, and the answer is nobody knows. We also don't know what it means to heart disease risk for these individuals because all the other major risk factors for heart disease and diabetes—metabolic syndrome, in short—improve."

– Gary Taubes

MOMENT OF CLARITY: "I don't think medical science has any idea why LDL-P would rise above 2,000 or even 3,000 in some people who eat a low-carb diet. But what I assume is that whatever positive role LDL plays in the health of these people, it's merely a sign they are improving by making the LDL work better. I don't see it as a bad thing."

– Dr. Fred Pescatore

Imagine this scenario: You switch your diet from the Standard American Diet over to a low-carb, high-fat diet to improve your health. After six months of eating this way, you've lost fifty pounds, raised your HDL cholesterol 25 points, dropped your triglycerides 100 points, and switched your LDL particle size from Pattern B to Pattern A. For all intents and purposes you are much healthier now than you were when you started. There's just one issue: Your LDL-C has shot up 100 points, taking your total cholesterol above 300. Plus, an NMR Lipoprofile test reveals that your LDL-P number has risen above 2,000. What the...?!

Most doctors who see LDL numbers like this automatically prescribe statin drugs without reservation. But if all your other cardio-metabolic health markers are extraordinarily good—including low triglycerides, high HDL cholesterol, normalized fasting blood sugar and insulin levels, and low CRP levels—how important are these numbers?

MOMENT OF CLARITY: "Here's the key question: If all your other health markers, including most of your lipid markers, are great eating a low-carbohydrate, high-fat diet, then are you at greater risk of heart disease if your LDL-P is high? All the population studies linking LDL-P to heart-health risks have been done in the context of people eating the Standard American Diet. So does it hold that because it's a good predictor in that context? Does it also apply to people eating low-carb, high-fat? Nobody knows the answer to this yet because the studies have not been conducted."

— Gary Taubes

MOMENT OF CLARITY: "If you're consuming a very low-carb, very high-fat diet, it's not unreasonable to think that you'll see a large increase in your LDL cholesterol. We've seen that happening even apart from the weight loss effect. How does this affect heart disease risk in the long run? We are not absolutely certain yet. If you improve everything and most of your cholesterol numbers look great but you have this big LDL cholesterol number, I think this is one of those big unknown questions that needs to be answered."

— Dr. Patty Siri-Tarino

I posed this question to another one of my experts for this book, Dr. Jeffry Gerber, a practicing physician in Denver, Colorado. He encourages his patients to follow a low-carb, high-fat diet because he believes it is healthier.

"In most patients who restrict carbohydrates in their diet we usually see all their cholesterol numbers go in the right direction," Dr. Gerber said. "But in a small percentage of people, LDL-C, total cholesterol, LDL-P, and ApoB [another key marker on the advanced cholesterol panel] might go up despite doing everything right in terms of nutrition. What do you do with patients like this? The bottom line is to watch them carefully. There are a lot of opinions about what to do about it, but I really think this area is unclear right now. That said, in the presence of low levels of inflammation and oxidative stress, perhaps these numbers have less meaning."

Despite the lack of conclusive evidence as to why this happens, Dr. Gerber said that he still challenges "the notion that low-carb dieters with high LDL-P or ApoB need to go on a statin drug. We just don't know the answer yet."

Dr. Rocky Patel, , another family doctor practicing medicine in Gilbert, Arizona, also prescribes low-carb diets for his patients. He, too, has noticed elevated LDL-P, LDL-C, and total cholesterol levels in some of the patients who begin reducing their carbohydrate consumption. When I asked him why, he answered frankly: "I don't know." But, he added, "If I had to come up with an educated guess, I would look at thyroid dysfunction as a possibility. If you down-regulate T3 and decrease the LDL receptor expression, then that could lead to excess lipoprotein expression. We know as a factor of heart attack risk that the standard thyroid stimulating hormone (TSH) levels will potentially put you at risk. If you look at most labs, the normal range can be from 0.4 to 4.5. But we know that if your TSH level is greater than 2.5, it can signal a higher risk of cardiovascular disease. I look at the overall thyroid function, examining T3 and T4."

Dr. Patel went on to explain the biggest problem with current research: "All of the LDL-P research that has been conducted so far is on a population eating the Standard American Diet. We don't have a study that looked at LDL-P with people who eat a low-carb diet. So, unfortunately, we really don't have the answer. When Paleo, primal, ketogenic, or low-carb patients come through my door, they get really worried when their lipid numbers come back very high. I don't have a lot of solid answers for them except to work them up and give them the options available."

MOMENT OF CLARITY: "For a low-carb dieter with a high LDL-P, LDL-C, and total cholesterol level in the presence of low triglycerides, high HDL-C, and low Small LDL-P values, I think that's a variant of the genes of deprivation. In a wild setting, someone with numbers like these would outsurvive other humans. If there was a three-week famine and others succumbed, these people would survive."

– Dr. William Davis

As you can see, the reasons for elevated cholesterol are multifaceted and can tend to overlap at times. Dr. Thomas Dayspring told me that people eating a low-carb, high-fat diet—sometimes referred to as a ketogenic diet (a topic we will address thoroughly in my next book *Keto Clarity*)—are in uncharted territory. "Currently we are noticing that in some people who eat a ketogenic diet with a lot of saturated fat there is a genetic threshold; when they exceed a certain amount of saturated fat intake, their liver starts producing cholesterol, leading to the formation of a lot of LDL particles," said Dr. Dayspring. "But it's because you have totally eliminated your insulin resistance and the metabolic mess associated with that. Is it possible that the arteries of these people could stand some extra LDL particles? Maybe, or maybe not. Until that is closely studied, we won't have an answer to that question."

MOMENT OF CLARITY: "If glucose and triglycerides stay low, there should not be a concern with rising cholesterol levels on a ketogenic diet. I don't know what's going on, but these reports may be associated with individuals consuming surplus calories in the form of fat or protein. If they are getting surplus calories from anywhere, then it will elevate blood fats. This is less dangerous than having chronically elevated blood glucose or chronic carbohydrate-induced spikes in glucose. You'll see CRP levels drop, triglycerides fall, HDL go up, and the size of the LDL particles get bigger."

– Dr. Dominic D'Agostino

In Dr. Gerber's opinion, worrying about high LDL-P levels if you are a low-carb dieter is much ado about nothing. "It may not be a significant issue at all," he told me. "In the absence of any evidence of plaque in the arteries, that's a great indicator that there isn't any risk at all." But, he added, "We're still interested in following patients like this to see what happens."

MOMENT OF CLARITY: "I myself have seen my LDL cholesterol go up from 150 to 190 and I don't feel as if I have a problem. It doesn't even worry me because my triglycerides are low, my HDL is high, and the ratio between the two is great. When I practiced in Hawaii, I had so many patients with a good, robust LDL cholesterol number and they were eighty or older. They had already outlived the average person, so how could I think that was a problem for them?"

– Dr. Cate Shanahan

If you are still worried about your high cholesterol level, the next chapter offers additional tests that are available to give you the peace of mind you are looking for about your heart health risks. But, as you can see, since the science is limited on this subject right now, there really is no clarity on this issue. We simply need better research and answers—much more than what Dr. Dayspring suggested, "just take the damn statin."

4. Familial Hypercholesterolemia (FH)

MOMENT OF CLARITY: "Familial hypercholesterolemia is a disease much more common than a lot of genetic diseases, but still relatively rare, compared with obesity and diabetes. People with FH have a problem with an LDL receptor; the liver isn't getting the message that there is a lot of cholesterol around, so it just keeps pumping it out. We know that those who carry one dose of the FH gene have a risk of heart attack in their twenties and thirties. If they are unlucky enough to have children with two doses of the FH genes, those children will die of heart attacks as teenagers."

– Dr. Ken Sikaris

A very small segment of the population suffers from a disease called FH, which is a genetic tendency for higher LDL cholesterol levels. FH is usually categorized as either homozygous familial hypercholesterolemia or heterozygous familial hypercholesterolemia. If you are one of the very rare one in a million people unlucky enough to have inherited homozygous FH from both parents, then cardiovascular disease is virtually inevitable at a very young age. But most people with this condition—one of out every five hundred people—have the more common form of heterozygous FH where they only received this genetic mutation from one parent.

MOMENT "Patients with familial hypercholesterolemia (FH) have a defect in
OF CLARITY: either the LDL receptor or the ApoB receptor. What you have to
understand is that lipoproteins floating around in your body is a good thing because they deliver nutrients and fat-soluble vitamins. We have to stop thinking of
cholesterol as a bad thing. Patients with FH have a tendency to build up LDL cholesterol and all the bad particles in the blood. If you're homozygous FH from both
your mother and your father, you actually don't live very long. A doctor can even
put them on statins and it wouldn't matter because they can't process LDL. The
heterozygous FH population from one parent affects only a small segment of the
population, and you can have a genetic test to see if you have this defect through
Athena Diagnostics."

– Dr. Jeffry Gerber

Perhaps you've noticed a notation regarding familial hypercholesterolemia on your cholesterol test results if your LDL or total cholesterol is
elevated. One of my regular blog readers sent me a note that she received
from her cardiologist via his nurse in response to her request for a CT Heart
Scan test to measure for any calcified plaque build-up in her arteries (more
on this in the next chapter). The doctor wanted to put her on a statin drug.
He also made an assumption about her cholesterol panel based solely on
her LDL and total cholesterol levels, which were 280 and 180, respectively:

*"Given how high your cholesterol (especially LDL, the bad kind) is, and
your family history, I suspect that you have an inherited form of hypercholesterolemia. I strongly recommend going back on a statin, at least at a low
dose. Lipitor is now generic, and you can try that instead of the statin. Many
insurance companies are not covering CTs and you may have to pay out of
pocket for that. I can order it, but you should also understand that it involves
a dose of radiation. If you have calcium deposits and STILL do not want to
go on a statin, then there is no real reason to get the study. An alternative
for statin-intolerant patients is apheresis, but since that is invasive, it would
make more sense to at least attempt statins again unless you really have a
contraindication."*

Unfortunately, this cardiologist's reaction is not out of the ordinary.
In fact, it's pretty indicative of the pessimistic attitude of many medical
professionals treating patients these days. Why did he automatically "sus-

pect" that this woman's total cholesterol and LDL numbers implied familial hypercholesterolemia? Why wouldn't he encourage her to have a more discriminating genetic test before jumping right to the conclusion that she has FH and thus needed to be taking a statin? Even worse is that he suggested that she go on the generic Lipitor "instead of the statin." Um, Lipitor *is* a statin, dude! Do doctors like this think we are all a bunch of uninformed idiots?

I was surprised the first time FH was indicated on my cholesterol test results. So when I decided to write *Cholesterol Clarity* I figured I'd take the plunge and get tested for it. Was my high total cholesterol that has been in excess of 400 at times due to FH or something else? In April 2013, I paid $1,200 to Ambry Genetics (Ambrygen.com/tests/familial-hypercholesterolemia) and the results would probably surprise the cardiologist whose note is reprinted above: According to my LDLR and ApoB genes, I have a "significantly decreased likelihood" of FH. Dr. Jeffry Gerber, who assisted me with getting this test run, confirmed that "the results are most favorable for you. May your LDL-P continue to rise and may you live a long and healthy life."

MOMENT OF CLARITY: "One-half of 1 percent of the population has familial hypercholesterolemia. But there have been studies showing that, even in those people, heart disease may not be as terrible as we thought."

– Dr. Donald Miller

It is possible to have total cholesterol levels of 300—even 400!—and not have heterozygous FH. People like this, myself included, may simply have difficulty clearing these LDL particles from their blood. I've said it before and I'll say it again: Elevated levels of cholesterol in the blood do not constitute a disease in and of itself. The cholesterol must penetrate the artery wall to cause any damage.

MOMENT OF CLARITY: "Cholesterol in the blood might correlate with heart disease in a population, but it can never be used by individual patients because of the propensity for discordance between cholesterol and atherogenic particle measurements. It takes cholesterol getting into the artery wall to kill you. And because all lipids—including cholesterol and triglycerides—are trafficked as passengers inside the lipoprotein, it's the type, the number, the quality of the lipoproteins that determine whether the little dump truck [lipoprotein] carrying the cholesterol molecules is going to invade your artery wall or not."

– Dr. Thomas Dayspring

MOMENT OF CLARITY: "There's no evidence at all that an isolated elevated biomarker justifies taking a statin. Quite frankly, I'm not bucking the system when I say that; even the statin guidelines don't call for treatment based on a singular biomarker, such as high total cholesterol—a fact that the drug manufacturers have in their recommendations regarding the use of statin medications."

– Dr. David Diamond

Some have suggested that people with FH should take a statin drug, but there are some simple changes in nutrition that can make a real difference. You can try switching from animal-based saturated fats to more plant-based monounsaturated sources like olive oil and avocados to see what impact that has at lowering your cholesterol levels. Additionally, you can prevent LDL particle oxidation and ensure proper thyroid care with iodine supplements and by adding antioxidants to your diet. Bottom line? Statin drugs are not inevitable even if you have FH.

5. Micronutrient Deficiencies

MOMENT OF CLARITY: "Obviously, micronutrient deficiency—particularly copper and iodine—could be factors in increased cholesterol levels. Oftentimes, we'll order a micronutrient panel and seek to correct those deficiencies through diet and supplementation."

– Dr. Rocky Patel

We need specific micronutrients to function at optimal levels. When our intake of these key vitamins and minerals is insufficient, our body may compensate by producing more LDL cholesterol particles. Paul Jaminet identified some of the most common micronutrient deficiencies he sees in people with higher levels of LDL cholesterol. "The major nutrient deficiencies leading to high LDL in some people are iodine, selenium, zinc, and copper," Jaminet told me. "Iodine and selenium are needed to make thyroid hormone and zinc and copper are necessary for making the body's most important extracellular antioxidant. If you don't have enough of that, then you'll have a lot of oxidative stress in the blood, which causes damage to your LDL and raises LDL levels."

Getting the proper micronutrients from your food and supplementing your diet when necessary can bring your LDL cholesterol levels back into line.

6. The Dangers of Chronic Bacterial Infection, Especially in the Teeth

MOMENT OF CLARITY: "Cholesterol is used to stabilize the tissue after an infection. All scars in the body are rich in cholesterol, including those in the arterial wall. In my view atherosclerotic lesions are just scars after previous infections."

– Dr. Uffe Ravnskov

Now that we know the purpose of cholesterol is to control inflammation and act as a healing agent, it makes sense that if there is an infection in your body your cholesterol will likely rise. In other words, if you have an underlying chronic bacterial infection, this could show up on your cholesterol test results as an elevated lipid panel. Conventional medicine immediately advises taking a statin drug to lower the cholesterol when it is higher than what is considered normal, but that ignores what has caused the cholesterol to go up in the first place—and it could be something in another part of your health you are completely unaware of and should pay closer attention to.

"The systemic infection that we see most often in my office is periodontal disease," Dr. Patel told me. "If we suspect that patients have an infection or gingivitis, we make sure they get a proper evaluation for bacterial load in the mouth. This could go undiagnosed for many years and be subclinical."

Unless your doctor or dentist is trained to look for this kind of thing, it could go completely unnoticed for many years, and meanwhile your cholesterol levels keep going up and up. This is nothing new to Dr. Ron Ehrlich, a holistic dentist practicing in Sydney, Australia. "Cholesterol is anti-inflammatory," Dr. Ehrlich said. "High cholesterol is not only an indicator that the body is defending against inflammation, but it may be the only indicator available in routine blood tests. High cholesterol in response to inflammation in tissues will naturally decrease once the cause of the inflammation is removed."

Once again, your family doctor will simply see that your cholesterol levels have gone up and recommend that you eat a low-fat diet, exercise more, and take a statin drug without ever investigating whether there is an underlying condition causing your elevated cholesterol levels. Dr. Ehrlich believes this issue is much more prevalent than people realize. "Periodontal disease is only one aspect of chronic dental infections," he said. "There are chronic infections at the apex of a tooth whose nerve has died. This does not need to be associated with pain. Similarly, there are chronic infections in jawbones associated with extracted teeth that may still harbor pathogens."

I have long suspected this is one of the reasons for my own high LDL and total cholesterol. When I was a sugar-addicted kid, I used to crunch hard candy and then leave it in there, completely oblivious to the damage it was causing to my teeth. Not surprisingly, I required four root canals and other major dental work in my twenties. The mercury amalgam fillings used to fill my teeth in the early 1990s, along with any infections at the site of those root canals, could certainly account for my elevated cholesterol levels. "Mercury is a heavy metal that can be a problem if it is constantly being released in the mouth from an old filling," Dr. Ehrlich said. "If there are dental mercury amalgams in someone's teeth, then it is stored in the kidney, liver, and brain, and to my mind would qualify as a heavy metal impacting your cholesterol."

There are other dentists, like Dr. Ehrlich, who are trained to look for these issues and they are worth consulting if you think this might be the cause of your own high cholesterol numbers. But isn't it fascinating to learn that something as seemingly unrelated to cholesterol as dental health might actually be the cause of your elevated levels? This makes the typical response of most doctors—to prescribe statins—seem even more knee-jerk and narrow-minded. Incidentally, in the midst of writing this book in June 2013, I was able to have all my mercury amalgams replaced with safer materials, as well as clean up several bacterial infections in my teeth. We'll see what impact this will have on my cholesterol levels as a result.

7. Stress

MOMENT OF CLARITY: "If you go back and look at why they determined that a raised LDL level is a risk factor for younger men only in the Framingham study, the answer to that is extremely clear. When people are stressed, their LDL levels go up. There was a study done in the 1960s looking at accountants. They found there were two times of the year when they were doing a lot of filing work, and during these periods their LDL levels rose an average of 60 percent, and then went down again after the stressful period subsided. If stress causes heart disease, stress causes LDL levels to go up, and we find LDL levels associated with higher rates of heart disease, don't you think it's the stress that is doing it? Wouldn't that be a possible hypothesis?"

— Dr. Malcolm Kendrick

Nobody reading this book ever experiences any stress; we all live such calm, relaxed lives. Yeah, right! The case could be made that we live in the most stressful period in the history of the world, and that can't come without consequences to your health, including having a direct effect on your cholesterol levels. Dr. Malcolm Kendrick, author of the book *The Great Cholesterol Con* and one of our featured experts in this book, is a well-known skeptic of the cholesterol-heart hypothesis. He told me that it is completely natural for a body under stress to produce more LDL cholesterol. "It's not that difficult to understand the concept that cholesterol in the body is used as a healing agent," he said. "Why would the body produce LDL? Well, LDL repairs damaged cells. It's a good thing in the short term when cortisol [known as the stress hormone] goes up during times of stress; that means all sorts of healthy, healing things are happening in the body. But in the long term, they are extremely unhealthy."

MOMENT OF CLARITY: "My plan for heart health includes lowering inflammation, lowering oxidative damage, lowering stress, and reducing sugar. Those are the four primary promoters of heart disease. But lowering stress is a tall order and encompasses many other activities that include community service, love, ending toxic relationships, volunteering, making love, playing with animals, and doing things that bring you joy. These are all important parts of heart health and health in general."

— Dr. Jonny Bowden

Dr. Kendrick added that allowing stress to continue to accumulate without a means of release forces the body to react as a way to protect itself. "What we're looking at here is a stress response," Dr. Kendrick explained. "It's the body getting itself ready for healing, fight and flight, all these things. Elevated LDL is part of that. And so there is a reasonably strong connection between increased LDL and heart disease. It doesn't mean that A caused B. It means that C caused A and B. How difficult can this be? It's like telling people that yellow fingers cause lung cancer."

MOMENT OF CLARITY: "I do think you should be concerned if you have high LDL or high total cholesterol, but the answer isn't to take medication to address the problem. Cholesterol levels can rise in response to consumption of too much sugar or in response to stress. Therefore, cholesterol serves as a biomarker of poor health conditions."

— Dr. David Diamond

So rather than prescribing that statin drug to lower your high cholesterol, why don't doctors recommend taking a yoga class, or finding time to take a walk with someone you love, or playing with your kids, or any number of other enjoyable, stress-relieving activities? Don't be surprised to see your cholesterol numbers come back to normal after you slow down and learn to decompress. As the kids might say, "Dude, take a chill pill!"

8. Hormonal Issues

MOMENT OF CLARITY: "Remember, a lot of things increase cholesterol, and when you understand how important cholesterol is you can easily see why. Stress increases it completely independent of diet. Your cholesterol goes up when you're fighting infections. Your HDL and LDL Pattern A go up when you eat saturated fat, but that's a good thing! And don't forget that the body needs cholesterol for the brain, for the cell membranes, and for the sex hormones—not to mention for vitamin D and bile acids."

— Dr. Jonny Bowden

Hormones: Ugh! Just the word can cause women to shudder. But as the hormones in a woman's body go up—during, say, menstruation or meno-pause—so goes her cholesterol. Taking birth control pills may also cause cholesterol levels to rise. And when a woman is pregnant, cholesterol is helping the baby's brain and body develop. That alone should prove that it is an essential substance of life!

MOMENT OF CLARITY: "If you're not metabolizing cholesterol, then you're not converting the cholesterol into all the stuff that it is there to be converted into, such as bile acids, which are necessary for digestion, sex hormones, blood pressure–regulating hormones, all the steroid hormones, etc. If you're blocking it [with a statin drug], then you are not doing all the good things you can do with cholesterol and making the LDL particle much more likely to become damaged."

— Dr. Chris Masterjohn

Polycystic ovarian syndrome (PCOS), a very clear sign of insulin resis-tance and metabolic syndrome, is another major cause of elevated LDL and reduced HDL cholesterol levels. This impaired glucose function can also increase small, dense LDL cholesterol particles, cause greater inflamma-tion, and promote a susceptibility to heart disease.

Men aren't totally off the hook, either: Andropause, also known as male menopause, can result in a precipitous increase in cholesterol levels. Stupid hormones!

The point is that cholesterol's response to changes in hormones is com-pletely normal and natural. If you get tested and your numbers are high, watch the trend over several readings to determine if the rise is caused by a temporary hormonal imbalance. When your doctor tries to push cholester-ol-lowering medications on you, tell him that you want to let the cholesterol do its thing: heal and protect your body.

MOMENT OF CLARITY: "The body never just throws away cholesterol. The body is very careful to preserve all its cholesterol because it is extremely valuable to the body."

— Stephanie Seneff

9. Weight Loss

Believe it or not, even when you are getting healthier by losing weight, your cholesterol levels can do some really funky things. LDL and total cholesterol may go up, HDL may go down, triglycerides may go up, blood sugar and blood pressure may rise. But relax: This is all a normal part of weight loss. Once you get the weight down to where you want it to be, and keep it stable, those cholesterol numbers will magically come back under control. That's why it's probably not a good idea to get your cholesterol tested while you are still actively losing weight. Reach your goal weight, become weight-stable for at least a month, and then get retested.

DOCTOR'S NOTE FROM DR. ERIC WESTMAN: One of the problems with measuring cholesterol levels in the blood is that they probably don't mean the same thing if you are losing weight. When the body is using its own fat energy storage for fuel, the blood cholesterol levels may shift dramatically and then return to their usual state when the weight loss has stopped. So if I am working with someone to lose weight, I don't worry about repeating the blood cholesterol levels until she has achieved her weight loss goal and become weight-stable.

Those are nine reasons why your cholesterol might be elevated. And guess what? We've just scratched the surface! We didn't even talk about other possible causes, like excessive exercise, fatty liver disease, and eating too little. But at least you can see how intricate and complicated the issue of cholesterol is—much more than your doctor will likely admit. At the very least, now you know why the knee-jerk reaction to push a statin medication to lower your cholesterol as the first line of defense without looking further into the cause is one of the most foolish things your doctor could ever do.

I'm sure there are some of you who, despite what you have read so far in this book, are *still* worried that high cholesterol numbers might be damaging your heart. Hey, I get it! The medical and health communities have been brainwashing you for decades. In the next chapter, you'll get more concrete ways for determining the real causes of high cholesterol, how concerned you need to be when your numbers rise, as well as tests for measuring whether any actual disease might be taking place.

KEY CHOLESTEROL CLARITY CONCEPTS

→ **Hypothyroidism can slow down the clearance of LDL cholesterol.**

→ **Carbohydrates increase triglycerides and Small LDL-P in the blood.**

→ **A low-carb, high-fat diet can increase LDL-P and total cholesterol in some people.**

→ **More research on the ketogenic diet is needed to learn the significance of cholesterol among people following this eating regimen.**

→ **Familial hypercholesterolemia is a genetic predisposition to have elevated cholesterol levels.**

→ **A lack of micronutrients, like iodine, selenium, zinc, and copper, raises cholesterol.**

→ **Certain causes of high cholesterol—including chronic bacterial infections, especially in the teeth—are often overlooked.**

→ **Stress raises cortisol levels, which manifests as higher cholesterol.**

→ **Hormones may cause cholesterol levels to fluctuate wildly.**

Chapter 15
I'm *Still* Worried about My High Cholesterol!

MOMENT OF CLARITY: "Among the vast majority of people, if their total cholesterol is between 160 and 240 mg/dL, the risk of early death is so minutely different that really there's nothing to be concerned with. If people have extremely high or extremely low cholesterol levels, then that's a slightly different discussion. About 98 percent of people have LDL and total cholesterol levels that are just fine."

– Dr. Malcolm Kendrick

MOMENT OF CLARITY: "I feel like a minister trying to convert people to my religion regarding what to really think about cholesterol."

– Dr. Cate Shanahan

I realize that some of you still have some lingering and nagging doubts in the back of your mind about everything you have learned in this book. This is completely normal: You're fighting against decades of misinformation, lies, and distortions of the truth that have been there all along. Old habits (and theories) die hard. I've certainly had my moments of doubt, given my own OMG cholesterol levels. Thankfully there are enough respected health experts—many of them featured in this book—who challenge the accepted wisdom of the day. Based on their cumulative decades of research and practice, here are ten things to consider before you freak out over your high cholesterol.

1. Determine whether your cholesterol really is high.
There's an automatic assumption that having LDL cholesterol over 100 or a total cholesterol level over 200 signals a greater risk of heart attack or stroke. But nutritional scientist and lipid expert Dr. Chris Masterjohn

asserts that these higher cholesterol numbers—which we have been told imply disease—do not match up with "nonmodernized populations that are totally free of heart disease."

"The best-studied population shown to be free of heart disease is the Kitavians of Papua, New Guinea," Dr. Masterjohn told me. "The males tend to have total cholesterol of around 180 mg/dL throughout their life. The females tend to have total cholesterol of 200 to 210 mg/dL when they are younger, but then it goes up to 250 mg/dL in middle age. As you can see, the males are within what we would say are the normal ranges of the 200 mg/dL cutoff. And yet the females have cholesterol levels in the area of what Americans would consider 'panic mode.'"

Panic mode is right. If a forty-seven-year-old woman in generally good health has a total cholesterol of 250, her doctor will be screaming for high-dose statin drugs and a low-fat diet. But the Kitavians prove that such fear is unfounded. In fact, Dr. Masterjohn notes that in Tokelau, New Zealand—where people routinely consume high amounts of coconut fat—total cholesterol levels for men increase from 180 to 220 mg/dL as they age, while women's levels jump from 200 to 245 mg/dL. Dr. Masterjohn believes that these are the numbers we should use as the guide for an ideal level of cholesterol: "My rough estimate about where to start looking for potential problems based on this data is that if total cholesterol gets over 220 for men or over 250 for women, then that's a possible indication that there might be a problem."

Dr. Masterjohn added that that there are other key numbers that need to be considered—that of HDL cholesterol level and the ratio of total-to-HDL cholesterol: "If a man has a total cholesterol of 250 and a total–to–HDL cholesterol ratio of 3, then I'm not too concerned. But if the ratio is around 7, that is often accompanied by metabolic problems that need to be looked into."

If your doctor looked at cholesterol levels through the prism of the Kitavians, a traditional culture free of heart disease, he might rethink what is popularly considered to be a high number.

2. Cholesterol reference ranges are an average of the population.

We just learned that the total cholesterol ranges in one heart-healthy population is higher than what mainstream medicine has told us is optimal.

But what about the conventional reference ranges that doctors are using to determine whether or not there is cause for concern? How reliable are those? If you ask Melbourne, Australia–based biochemist Dr. Ken Sikaris, he'd tell you that those cutoff points for measuring cholesterol are merely an average of the population being tested. They do not, therefore, indicate whether *you* are in a potentially diseased state.

"The interpretation of the cholesterol numbers is in itself a self-fulfilling prophecy," Dr. Sikaris explained. "People looked at cholesterol levels and if they were at a certain cutoff point, then the risk of a heart attack increased. If you look at what that cutoff point means, it's nothing more than the average cholesterol in that population. So if your cholesterol is above average, then your heart disease risk is above average. But that cutoff point threshold is really right smack in the middle of the general population."

Furthermore, Dr. Sikaris believes that the recommendation to keep total cholesterol levels below 200 is not only arbitrary and unrealistic, it runs counter to how most lab tests are done. "With cholesterol, if you're above the average, then it's concluded you've got an increased risk of the disease," Dr. Sikaris said. "We've lowered the cutoff so that it is so sensitive to disease that the poor patients who fall outside the range think they have some sort of terrible mutation that requires them to do something drastic."

By *something drastic*, Dr. Sikaris is referring to resorting to statin drug treatment and cutting fat and calories from your diet. But, as he pointed out to me, these are overreactions to a problem that doesn't really exist: "When you tell people that 50 percent of the population has levels above that point, they start to relax and wonder about risk factors other than total cholesterol. As you can see, it's all sort of self-reinforcing the cholesterol myths. I suppose that's when the food industry got on board and started labeling everything 'low cholesterol.'"

Keep this in mind—it's a critical point: The measuring stick of 200 for your total cholesterol levels is merely the average of the population tested, so being above that level doesn't automatically put you at risk for anything.

3. Cutting dietary fat and cholesterol will not improve your health.

We've talked a lot about the surprising role dietary fat—especially saturated fat—and cholesterol play in *improving* heart health. This runs counter to what most people have been raised to believe, as Minneapolis-based registered dietitian Cassie Bjork (aka "Dietitian Cassie") discovered in her work with clients. Bjork told me that it can be "very shocking" to people when they learn that eating fat and cholesterol doesn't make you fat and clog your arteries as we have been led to believe. "There is simply no sound science behind the prevention message that reducing saturated fat in your diet will lower your risk of heart disease," she said. "Science is actually showing the opposite effect, and health educators need to stop teaching outdated, non-research-based information."

If you are worried about your high cholesterol levels, Bjork suggests that you look at the breakdown of your LDL particles using advanced cholesterol screening (as discussed in chapter 9). These will show you the benefits that result from adding more fat and cholesterol to your diet. "My favorite advanced cholesterol test is the NMR Lipoprofile because it shows you the difference in your LDL particles," she said. "Most people only see their total cholesterol, LDL, and HDL when their doctor tests their blood."

Bjork told me that without the proper context of all the other factors covered in this book, the total cholesterol number tells her "pretty much nothing" about someone's state of health. It's good to know that there are people working in the nutrition and medical communities who know and are sharing the truth.

4. The risk from statins outweighs the absolute risks of having a heart attack.

Chapter 5 went over the many health risks associated with taking statin drugs. But there are other startling statistics worth sharing, especially since tens of millions of people are taking these drugs in an effort to improve their health. Researcher and physician Dr. Uffe Ravnskov has been sounding the antistatin alarm for some time. "The benefit you receive from statin treatment is trivial," he told me. "For a sixty-five-year-old man who has had a heart attack, the chance of being alive for another five years is about 90 percent. By taking a statin every day, he increases those odds by only 2 percent. That's all."

Pharmaceutical industry spokespeople would have us believe that the benefits of taking their drugs are far more dramatic. But they're merely pointing out *relative* risks, which show a greater percentage of *perceived* benefit, not *absolute* risks, which have a far less significant benefit. "The drug companies tell us that we can lower the risk of a heart attack by 20 percent with statins because of the 2 percent difference in mortality rates," Dr. Ravnskov explained. "With a statin, it's 8 percent and without statin treatment it's 10 percent. But to use the change in percentage rather than percentage points is incredibly misleading."

According to Dr. Ravnskov, there is a minuscule increase of two percentage points in your survival if you take a statin. But here's the negative trade-off, based on independent research: Statin drugs also *increase* the risk of diabetes by 4 percent, impotence by 20 percent, and muscle and joint pain by upwards of 40 percent. I don't know about you, but in my opinion the potential downsides of high cholesterol simply pale in comparison to these very serious side effects.

There is also emerging evidence now that statin treatment may cause cancer, Dr. Ravnskov warned. "A relevant question is this: Do you want to potentially die from having a heart attack or do you want to die from the cancer your cholesterol-lowering medication induced?"

5. Consider your gut health.

Chapter 14 offered nine reasons why your cholesterol levels might be elevated. Here's another one worth looking into: The problem could be parasites or protozoa in your gut. Ewwww! Paul Jaminet recommends getting the Metametrix GI Effects stool test, which locates any microscopic bugs that may be wreaking havoc in your intestines or bowels. Learn more about this test at Metametrix.com.

6. Try improving your numbers
with cholesterol-modifying supplements.

Rather than prescription drugs, one of the experts quoted in this book and board-certified nutritionist Dr. Jonny Bowden recommends a series of cholesterol-modifying supplements that have proved highly effective at improving lipid panels and overall cardiovascular health. "My top supplements for heart health are omega-3s from fish oil, magnesium, coenzyme Q10, resveratrol, curcumin, vitamin D, vitamin C, and citrus bergamot," said Dr. Bowden. "These supplements have anti-inflammatory action, antioxidant power, and they help support the arteries and heart health in many other ways. Citrus bergamot lowers blood sugar, as does magnesium; it also lowers triglycerides and raises HDL cholesterol. Magnesium relaxes the artery walls while lowering blood pressure."

It bears repeating: Your body does not have a statin deficiency! Instead, it craves the actual nutrients necessary to protect itself, no matter what your cholesterol level is. "Give the body what it needs and it will function the way it's supposed to," Dr. Bowden concluded.

7. Consider a CT heart calcium scan of your heart.

MOMENT OF CLARITY: "There is one test that is slightly controversial that I really like to run. It's called the CT heart scan because it goes right down to see if there is any plaque there in your arteries. If it comes back zero, then you're good. If you find plaque in one of your arteries, there's usually plaque formation somewhere else in the body. Chelation therapy has been shown to reverse plaque and minimize cardiac damage after a myocardial infarction."

– Dr. Fred Pescatore

Here's a question I had and you might have, too: Does high cholesterol actually damage the heart? The complicated answer is that elevated cholesterol in and of itself is not a disease. The problem comes from oxidized LDL particles penetrating the arterial wall and turning into calcified plaque. This is why I encourage anyone worried about high cholesterol levels to get a CT heart calcium scan of their chest, which will show if there's any calcium build-up happening in their arteries. Cardiac surgery professor Dr. Donald Miller agreed that this simple, noninvasive test is "a fairly reasonable" way to determine whether there is any "actual disease in your coronary arteries. If the score is low," said Dr. Miller, "then you can forget about high cholesterol meaning anything. If the score is high, then making appropriate changes by consuming a low-carbohydrate diet will be necessary."

As someone who has had high cholesterol for many years, I've paid close attention to my CT heart scan calcium scores. In preparation for this book, I had this test done in 2009 and again in 2013. Both times my cholesterol was in excess of 350 and both times my CT heart calcium scan score came back as zero. Dr. Miller said it can be "very comforting" to people like me who have high cholesterol levels to see a low or zero CT heart calcium scan score. "If you don't have any calcium in your coronary arteries, then quit measuring your cholesterol," he said. "A good CT heart scan calcium score means your risk of coronary artery disease is extremely low. Go on about your business and worry about something else."

The CT heart scan calcium score test is relatively inexpensive (it costs less than $100 in South Carolina, where I live) and must be ordered by your doctor. Just make sure your doctor orders the right one; there's a similar test where dye is shot through your body that can cost hundreds of dollars more. Here's a link to a YouTube video of my wife Christine getting a CT heart scan: http://youtu.be/XeAhhWn2h_Q.

Dr. Ronald Krauss, senior scientist and director of atherosclerosis research at Children's Hospital Oakland Research Institute, is another doctor who recommends knowing your coronary calcium score from a CT heart scan, which he considers "the most well documented indicator of risk of a heart attack. It can be useful in helping to decide what treatment, if any, is necessary," said Dr. Krauss. "If somebody's calcium score came back negative, then I'd likely be less aggressive than if there was a positive result, and vice versa."

The good news is that if your CT heart scan calcium score comes back as zero, you don't need to have it tested again for five to seven years. For people dealing with high cholesterol, this simple and painless three-minute test is an excellent way to determine whether you actually have signs of heart disease or not.

8. A carotid IMT test also measures the presence of plaque.

There's another neat way to measure for any signs of heart disease: the carotid intima media thickness (IMT) test, which uses ultrasound to measure the thickness around your carotid artery. Dr. Jeffry Gerber uses this test in conjunction with the CT heart scan. "It takes thirty or more years to develop plaque," Dr. Gerber noted. "For patients with elevated cholesterol levels, you can run their cholesterol profile every three to four months to see how they are doing."

MOMENT OF CLARITY: "Doing a carotid IMT ultrasound can give you an actual measure of atherosclerosis."

— Dr. Patty Siri-Tarino

All this testing can give you peace of mind, in addition to alerting your doctor to potential damage. But Dr. Gerber says you can go one step further. "If patients are especially concerned, I've had them get heart catheterizations. But that's only for patients who are really at great risk based on their test results."

It's good to know that there are multiple ways to determine if there is actual damage to your heart. If you're worried, get these tests done and go from there.

DOCTOR'S NOTE FROM DR. ERIC WESTMAN: Imagine back to when Columbus left Spain and headed toward the New World, despite the outcry that he would fall off the edge of the world. Was there someone at the top of the mast looking ahead to be sure to turn around if and when the end of the world was spotted? Despite the outcry from people that eating low-carb is harmful, there is no evidence to support this belief. But, if you want, get your arteries checked to see if you have atherosclerosis to be absolutely sure. The reason doctors check blood cholesterol to begin with is to monitor and prevent disease in your arteries.

9. Engage in regular periods of intermittent fasting to lower LDL particles.

Wait, did you just say fasting? As in not consuming any food at all for a period of time? Yep, sure did. The idea of fasting turns a lot of people off. But according to Dr. William Davis—author of the *New York Times* bestselling book *Wheat Belly*—regular, intermittent fasting has been shown to lower the level of LDL particles in your blood. "My anecdotal experience has shown me that people with exaggerated LDL values benefit more than most by doing such things as intermittent fasting, which mimics the natural human experience of deprivation," said Dr. Davis, who practices in Milwaukee. "When you are doing intermittent fasting, you might see a rise in triglycerides for several days afterwards. This is a good thing because those are triglycerides that are released from stored body fat. That's a totally natural response. People sometimes get upset when they've lost a good deal of weight very quickly and their triglycerides go up, the HDL goes down, and blood sugar goes up. They mistakenly think the diet hurt them, but this is the expected change that comes with weight loss and all the numbers subside and look much better several weeks later after the patient becomes weight-stable."

Dr. Davis realizes that eating sporadically for long periods of time like our prehistoric ancestors is perhaps too unrealistic in modern society. But we do have the genetic ability to handle regular periods of fasting. "In 2013, there are very few people who have to tell their families they're not going to be able to eat for another two weeks," Dr. Davis said. "Our ancestors may have survived on a squirrel for days. As a result, we have genes that allow us to tolerate periods of deprivation."

Intermittent fasting might not be your first choice, but it's certainly something worth considering if high cholesterol is putting you in harm's way.

10. Reverse insulin resistance by lowering fasting blood sugar and insulin.

One of the most critical aspects of our health rarely gets discussed in connection with heart disease: insulin resistance. This is a key metabolic state, when cells stop responding properly to the hormone insulin, and it can make you more susceptible to heart disease. Dr. Malcolm Kendrick considers the fasting insulin level to be "the most important health marker. It will tell you virtually everything you need to know about your health."

And he's not alone. Dr. Rocky Patel regularly employs out-of-the-box data to "determine the best course of treatment, if necessary. So I'm not just looking at cholesterol numbers," he told me, "I'm looking at all the other stuff, too. Quite frankly, based on my experience dealing with elevated lipids in the presence of controlled insulin resistance and inflammation, the real question becomes whether we should even care about cholesterol. Unfortunately, we don't have a real clear answer to this yet."

The science may not be conclusive, but there is enough evidence to suggest that getting insulin resistance under control is integral to heart and overall health. In the next chapter, we take a closer look at the cholesterol guidelines being used by your primary care doctor. Are they grounded in solid science? If you've been soaking in everything you have been reading up until now, then you probably know the answer.

MOMENT OF CLARITY: "I wish a lot more people would stop paying attention to their cholesterol numbers and start paying attention to what they are putting into their bodies. You can always manipulate statistics and numbers, but in the end it just comes down to common sense. Does it seem like you feel good? Does it seem like the food you are eating is truly natural? So what are you worried about if your LDL is elevated within that context? What are you trying to prove? Are you just looking to have something to say when someone asks you what your numbers are?"

— Dr. Cate Shanahan

KEY CHOLESTEROL CLARITY CONCEPTS

→ **Traditional populations with no heart disease have healthy cholesterol levels, which are often higher than the baselines for Western societies.**

→ **Cholesterol reference ranges are merely an average of the general population.**

→ **Cutting dietary fat and cholesterol will not improve your health.**

→ **Health improvements from statins are minimal, while risks are great.**

→ **Test your gut microbiota for cholesterol-raising bugs.**

→ **Basic supplements to your diet can alter cholesterol numbers.**

→ **Get a CT calcium scan or carotid IMT to determine plaque in your coronary arteries.**

→ **Regular periods of intermittent fasting may lower LDL particle levels.**

→ **To truly make a difference in your heart health, reverse insulin resistance.**

Chapter 16

But Aren't the Cholesterol Guidelines Based on Solid Science?

(M)OMENT OF CLARITY: "Research money is drying up and making it difficult to study this cholesterol issue further."

– Dr. Fred Kummerow

If the cholesterol guidelines used by most doctors aren't backed up by comprehensive, thorough, or up-to-date research, as we've discussed, how is it that patients and their doctors have come to place so much faith in them? That's a fair question to ask.

(M)OMENT OF CLARITY: "The gold standard in research is the randomized, controlled clinical trial and until you prove something in this setting you cannot state that something is based on science. Meanwhile, everybody has got to eat something and everybody is trying to do the best they can given their fondness for various foods and how their bodies respond to those foods. People want to know what they can do about their personal health while they are waiting for the research to give them better guidance."

– Dr. Patty Siri-Tarino

The ATP Guidelines Attempt to Set Standards for Cholesterol Treatment

Most people outside the medical profession don't even realize that cholesterol level guidelines exist. But they do: The Adult Treatment Panel (ATP) Guidelines are provided to doctors by the National Cholesterol Education Program at the National Institutes of Health. The latest edition, ATP III, was published in 2002, and you can view these guidelines at nhlbi.nih.gov/guidelines/cholesterol.

MOMENT OF CLARITY: "There's such inertia with all the cholesterol guidelines, especially with such a big moneymaking industry producing the statin drugs. People are unwilling to address it because it would have such a huge impact. We've been trying hard for the past twenty years not to label half the population at risk for heart disease. But the committees that determine cholesterol cutoff points are concerned about having to treat half the population when the health system can't afford that burden. We need to make this manageable and affordable for the health system to handle."

– Dr. Ken Sikaris

The self-described purpose of the ATP Guidelines is "detection, evaluation, and treatment of high blood cholesterol in adults." The NIH makes it sound so official and authoritative! But then so does the U.S. Department of Agriculture (USDA), which brags that its Dietary Guidelines for Americans (the basis for MyPlate) offers the perfect way to eat. Don't get me started on that one. Let's just say that, in both these cases, the intentions may have been good, but the execution was utterly horrible.

MOMENT OF CLARITY: "The problem with this science field is you can speculate about virtually anything and then find data to support or refute it."

– Gary Taubes

There's a long list of MDs, PhDs, and RDs cited in the ATP III Guidelines Executive Summary report. These "experts" are meant to lend legitimacy to the views expressed in the report—views that are the final word on treating patients with high cholesterol in the United States. Based on these guidelines, here are a few of the recommendations doctors are expected to follow in treating the cholesterol levels of their patients:

- ► LDL cholesterol levels should be below 100 mg/dL.
- ► LDL cholesterol is the "primary target of cholesterol-lowering therapy."
- ► HDL cholesterol levels should be above 40 mg/dL.
- ► Total cholesterol levels below 200 mg/dL are "desirable."
- ► As statin drugs become cheaper, more people should be taking them.
- ► Reducing consumption of saturated fat and cholesterol is imperative.

- ► Carbohydrates should comprise 50–60 percent of your daily calories.
- ► Increasing physical activity and managing weight are important.
- ► Get a referral to see a dietitian for more guidance on nutrition.

It's infuriating. Here we have what is considered the gospel truth about cholesterol that is supposedly based on sound, comprehensive research. Except that it's not. But why rock the boat, right? That seems to be the overriding fallback philosophy of our medical community and government. Trouble is, they are fooling around with our health in the process.

MOMENT OF CLARITY: "Wherever you look, it's just so obvious that these messages are just completely wrong and there's no evidence whatsoever to support them. But it's amazing how powerfully they've been incorporated into the subconscious of humanity."

— Dr. Malcolm Kendrick

MOMENT OF CLARITY: "They consistently misquote a study by Ancel Keys, which doesn't distinguish between total cholesterol variations. But this continues to show up in very important literature like the ATP III Cholesterol Guidelines. These are supposed to be the bedrock of guidelines about cholesterol, and if you question this at a medical meeting, the doctors are all going to turn and throw stones at you. This is what the drug companies are using when they say to doctors, 'You have to get somebody's total cholesterol number down.' But it's based largely on all this old data that has not been analyzed properly."

— Dr. Cate Shanahan

The ATP IV Guidelines Are Not Likely to Change for the Better

Several of the experts interviewed for this book are quite pessimistic about the forthcoming ATP IV Guidelines, expected to be released sometime in 2014. In fact, Dr. Ronald Krauss, who has been researching the relevance of LDL particle testing, says a shift to making only "evidence-based" recommendations means the new guidelines may have hit a major roadblock. "They've been struggling with getting evidence-based research for recommendations that can be used for lipid management," he told me. "Part of the problem is that the guidelines process requires a level of evidence that is often difficult if not impossible to achieve in clinical settings."

Dr. Krauss noted that it is a "huge challenge to develop evidence-based guidelines because nobody is going to do a study that tests the effect that a certain nutrient has on heart disease outcomes, particularly in the general population. It's almost impossibly time-consuming and expensive."

As a result, much of the research is years away from being fully vetted. "The people [creating the ATP Guidelines] are being careful about stepping ahead of really firm evidence, but what they don't realize is that some of us have been stepping ahead of the evidence all this time," Dr. Krauss said. "You go with the best information you have."

Dr. Krauss admitted that part of the challenge is that new data can disrupt common practice, which can undermine the credibility of the medical community. But that is an integral and necessary part of science. "We sometimes change our minds and we need to be able to do so," he said. "Otherwise, you're never going to learn anything."

MOMENT OF CLARITY: "There are ads being run in *Science* magazine luring new scientists to other countries since most of the funding for heart disease has dried up in the United States. I used to have support for my work at the rate of $200,000 a year. For the last three years, I had to use $175,000 of my own money to keep the two people I have working in my lab. I'm having a really hard time getting funded."

— Dr. Fred Kummerow

Dr. Thomas Dayspring agreed that the process will be slow. "The ATP IV Cholesterol Guidelines aren't coming any time soon," he said. "They're still under review by the National Heart, Lung and Blood Institute. Once those people sign off on it, it's going to go off to experts around the country for so-called public comment and then eventually it will get published."

Unfortunately, when the guidelines do finally make it into print, Dr. Dayspring believes they will be useless because "They can only recommend things that have what's called Level 1 evidence, and that means anything tested with prospective large, randomized, blind clinical trials." Unfortunately, not many of those comprehensive trials exist. "Lab measurements such as ApoB, LDL-P, and non-HDL cholesterol have not been tested like this and nobody is ever going to do these trials," Dr. Dayspring lamented. "When they did these trials on cholesterol markers twenty years ago, it was all on LDL-C, and thus it is the only marker that has the Level 1 evidence."

MOMENT OF CLARITY: "The institutional pressures and the liability pressures are great. We're on this thing for evidence-based medicine now, and we're basically dumbing it down to treating numbers. So most physicians don't put very much thought into it anymore. They're busy in their practice and they don't want to get into trouble."

— Dr. Dwight Lundell

Dr. Dayspring told me to expect the focus on lowering the LDL-C number to become even more intense. "Many people doubt that the new guidelines are going to say much more than 'If your cholesterol is high, take a statin and be done with it.' It's pathetic."

New York City family physician Dr. Fred Pescatore, who emphasizes nutritional medicine, agrees with Dr. Dayspring. He, too, is disappointed by the continued focus on LDL-C as the primary treatment modality for elevated cholesterol levels. "The newest recommendation that is going to come out in the ATP IV Cholesterol Guidelines is that they will want your LDL-C to be below 70," he said. "I think all that's going to do is kill people. It will show up as death rates going up."

Dr. Pescatore believes that there is only one logical and insidious reason for the LDL-C focus: "The only reason the whole cholesterol myth exists is because we have a drug to treat it. Therefore, if we have a drug, why not use it? The pharmaceutical companies have convinced the entire world that they need to be on a statin drug simply because the drug was made."

Dr. Rocky Patel told me that the new Affordable Care Act healthcare law, which goes into full effect in 2014, will require doctors to "be held more accountable," not just for the health of their patients but for the costs involved in providing that care. "The ATP III Cholesterol Guidelines took into account the cost of testing versus the benefit to the patient. That's one of the reasons why advanced lipid testing may not be recommended in the ATP IV Cholesterol Guidelines—because they can be expensive to do."

In a perfect world, doctors and patients would be given cholesterol guidelines (and dietary guidelines, for that matter) based on sound and current science. But that is unlikely to happen. And as long as statin drugs are big business, the government and medical community are unlikely to move away from the status quo, or invest in research that might disprove the cholesterol-heart hypothesis. As a result, it is unlikely that the ATP IV Cholesterol Guidelines will be anything close to the last word—not by a long shot!

Coming up in the next chapter: We look at why the low-fat, vegetarian diets that are glorified for improving cholesterol and being "heart healthy" may not be everything they're cracked up to be.

KEY CHOLESTEROL CLARITY CONCEPTS

→ **Many people think cholesterol recommendations are backed by sound scientific research.**

→ **The ATP Guidelines draw on the top medical and research professionals.**

→ **The ATP III Guidelines, published in 2002, focus on LDL-C as a primary marker of heart disease.**

→ **ATP IV Guidelines, expected to come in 2014, will only accept Level 1 evidence**

→ **Obtaining "evidence-based" recommendations is impossible to achieve.**

→ **Advanced cholesterol testing will never be adequately researched.**

→ **The continued focus on LDL-C will simply be used to market statin drugs.**

→ **Stop having your cholesterol tested unless you're still worried that it matters.**

Chapter 17

The Low-Fat, Vegetarian Myth

MOMENT OF CLARITY: "How do you break people from thinking *low-fat* means "healthy"? In the end, the truth will prevail. Eventually, the real message is going to win out. The only way you can suppress the truth is with vast amounts of money and effort. That is exactly what we are seeing happen right now. At some point, though, that will diminish because the evidence is utterly conclusive and it all goes in one direction. I see this thinking on fat and cholesterol to be a bit like communism. It lasted for fifty years and was sustained by people telling lies for fifty years. Eventually, people recognized that this system just didn't work."

— Dr. Malcolm Kendrick

When you think about a "heart-healthy" diet, it's almost impossible to get away from the low-fat, vegetarian approach. For millions of people, they think that is the only way to go. But that only makes sense if you mistakenly believe that consuming foods rich in saturated fat will raise your LDL cholesterol and lead to heart disease. But you don't believe that anymore, do you?

MOMENT OF CLARITY: "Fat is not the issue and it is never going to be an issue. Eating fat and cholesterol does not necessarily raise your cholesterol levels. Eating healthy fats from real whole food sources is perfectly fine. Eliminating artificial foods like sugar, white bread, and white pasta will actually keep your cholesterol right where it is supposed to be."

— Dr. Fred Pescatore

If you are currently eating a low-fat, vegetarian diet and all of your cholesterol numbers and other key health markers (blood sugar, insulin, C-reactive protein, etc.) are absolutely perfect, then why would you ever change it? I'm the first person to cheer people on if they have found a nutritional plan that keeps them happy and healthy. But I would also point out that, after decades of demonizing saturated fat and cholesterol, it might be hard for such a person to recognize what is becoming an irrefutable fact: that eliminating fat and cholesterol from your diet could be doing more harm than good.

MOMENT OF CLARITY: "If you're on a low-fat diet, you can underpopulate the LDL particles with the proper amounts of fat. Small, dense LDL particles tend to be associated with various health problems. And low HDL cholesterol levels happen when someone is eating this way. One reason their HDL becomes too low is they are not consuming enough saturated fat in their diet."

– Paul Jaminet

We have discussed this point at length, but it is worth echoing again and again: Every cell in your body needs cholesterol to function properly. When you deprive your body of essential nutrients like saturated fat and dietary cholesterol and then replace them with carbohydrate sources of energy (whole grains, sugary fruits, starchy vegetables), the body responds by making more triglycerides, reducing the level of HDL cholesterol, and creating more of those nasty small, dense LDL particles. This triple threat of health markers is unavoidable when your diet is primarily high-carb, low-fat, and vegetarian.

MOMENT OF CLARITY: "If you eat a low-saturated-fat, high-carb diet, it tends to raise Lipoprotein(a). This is yet another example of why low-fat is not the answer to cardiovascular risk."

– Dr. Ronald Krauss

The Low-Fat, Vegetarian Diet Is All about Lowering LDL Cholesterol

Stop and think about it for a moment. Why did the low-fat, vegetarian diet become such a popular option for lowering cholesterol levels? And why is it commonly thought to promote good heart health? It goes hand in hand with the cholesterol-heart hypothesis and the emphasis on two numbers: your LDL-C and total cholesterol. When demonstrable evidence showed that you could lower those two numbers simply by cutting saturated fat and cholesterol—found most commonly in animal-based foods—out of your diet, the simultaneous demonization of fat, cholesterol, and meat, along with the celebration of carbohydrate-based foods, began in full force.

Of course, after reading this book you know better now; the body is way too complicated to respond to just two arbitrary numbers on your cholesterol panel. But doctors have been drinking the cholesterol hypothesis Kool-Aid for decades, so they still get excited by an LDL cholesterol level of 65 and total cholesterol of 101. So what if the patient's HDL is 23, or their triglycerides are 227, or (if they even bothered to do advanced cholesterol testing) all their LDL particles are small and dense? Can you see how easily a low-fat diet and statin drug combo therapy might become the go-to treatment for high cholesterol?

MOMENT OF CLARITY: "What complicates the diet story is the simple fact that statins lower LDL cholesterol and save lives, at least in some patient populations. This has driven the belief that anything that lowers LDL cholesterol must be a good thing, and since saturated fat raises LDL cholesterol, it must be a bad thing. Even the drug companies push this, by mixing diet and drugs in their commercials. If you can't lower your cholesterol enough by avoiding butter, cheese, and red meat, then go for our statins."

— Gary Taubes

Dean Ornish's Low-Fat, Vegetarian Diet Trial Never Isolated Nutrition

Dr. Dean Ornish is one of the leading voices of the low-fat, vegetarian movement. He became famous for his Lifestyle Heart Trial, a series of clinical research trials that attempted to reverse the progression of coronary artery disease through lifestyle changes like exercise, stress management, smoking cessation, and a low-fat, vegetarian diet. The results have been published in some pretty prestigious medical journals, including *Lancet* and the *Journal of the American Medical Association*, and Dr. Ornish is fond of saying that his approach is the only one that has been proven to reverse heart disease. He said that repeatedly, in fact, when I interviewed him on my *The Livin' La Vida Low-Carb Show* podcast in 2008.

But several of the experts I interviewed for this book question his claims, including Dr. William Davis, a cardiologist who believes that the Lifestyle Heart Trial results are incredibly misleading. The study was "a very teensy, weensy trial" of a nutritional plan, he told me. Furthermore, "We know that of the less than thirty high-risk patients who started on his Lifestyle Heart Program, something like twenty-eight out of the thirty people in the five-year period of his program ended up having a heart attack, a heart procedure, or some other hospitalization. In other words, these were not twenty-eight people who were walking around, happy and dancing, eating a healthy diet. These were people who had very, very serious problems during their five years in this trial."

Dr. Davis also questions Dr. Ornish's primitive methodology for measuring heart disease. "The participants did have less progression of disease, but using a very crude measure, something called QCA or quantitative coronary angiography. This is not a good way to assess the burden of disease." According to Dr. Davis, variables like these make the study's conclusions shortsighted. "I think what he showed was that his very low-fat diet, along with the entire lifestyle package, achieved normalization of endothelial function. All that means is that he allowed the arteries of his study participants to relax, and that gives them an apparent increase in the diameter of the blood vessel and a decrease in the percent of blockage."

The starker reality, added Dr. Davis, is that Dr. Ornish "did not eliminate cardiovascular events from happening" in the patients who participated in his study. "These study patients had many cardiovascular events," he added. "So we've got to be careful about drawing any conclusions from this study."

But Dr. Ornish's study got a whole lot of people who were worried about their high cholesterol levels leading to heart disease to switch to a low-fat, vegetarian diet. And yet how does that impact overall health? "I think there is a benefit if that [heart disease] is your only metric," said Dr. Davis. "But if we ask if this truly is the ideal diet that represents what humans are evolutionarily adapted to consume, the diet that minimizes all the diseases we have control over, then I would say absolutely not."

In fact, Dr. Davis considers the low-fat, vegetarian diet "an anti-evolutionary interpretation of how humans should live." Worse, he added, it can lead to "multiple metabolic distortions and health problems." It's better than eating crap fast food and all that, but it certainly ain't the ideal way to eat.

DOCTOR'S NOTE FROM DR. ERIC WESTMAN: Recent independent research has shown that in some people the ultra–low–fat diet worsens the LDL profile, and exercise only partially reduces this effect. So it is important to see how whatever lifestyle you choose affects your health, and not just take someone else's word for it.

What is sometimes forgotten about the Lifestyle Heart Trial is that it was not just about diet, says cognitive neuroscience professor Dr. David Diamond, though diet is what the trial ultimately became most famous for. But the lifestyle changes implemented were equally important. Unfortunately, what got picked up by the media and marketed to the public was that to be healthy you need to cut fat and eat more plant-based foods. The truth is the low-fat, vegetarian diet has never ever been isolated in any study.

"The most high-profile diet guru emphasizing a diet low in fat, high in fruits and vegetables, with only a small amount of lean meat is Dean Ornish, and he promotes the use of this diet as a treatment for heart disease," Dr. Diamond told me. "Ornish claims his diet recommendations lower cholesterol in the blood and improve health, but he's never actually conducted a study manipulating *only* diet."

In other words, improvements to health may have occurred regardless of the diet plan, and this is an important distinction. "In Dr. Ornish's research, people reduced their smoking, cut down on their stress, increased exercise, and, oh, by the way, they also happened to reduce their saturated fat and cholesterol as well," says Dr. Diamond. "The critical question is if all those lifestyle changes are having the desired effect, perhaps even despite the diet."

Low-fat, vegetarian advocates like Dr. Ornish may be "on the right track with their lifestyle recommendations," Dr. Diamond added, even if their diet advice falls short of the mark for a lot of people.

"People need to realize that good health isn't in a pill. Changes in lifestyle, such as smoking cessation, reducing consumption of sugar, stress control, and exercise, in conjunction with eating natural fats, including butter, with full-fat cheese, grass-fed beef, nuts, vegetables, and dark chocolate, are the best prescription for great health," Dr. Diamond added.

The Egg Whites Fallacy

One of the worst trends in what is supposed to be healthy eating is what has happened to eggs—specifically the vilification of the incredibly nutritious yolks. Many popular restaurant chains are lauding their new egg white sandwiches promoted to consumers as a more healthy option. In 2012, Subway introduced a new "healthy" menu item with their Black Forest Egg White And Cheese Flatbread Morning Melt breakfast sandwich; then in 2013, McDonald's introduced their much-heralded Egg White Delight McMuffin as a "lighter" option. Expect to see even more egg white menu offerings in restaurants as long as people continue to fear the consumption of saturated fat and cholesterol. This is further evidence of just how deeply entrenched this demonization of dietary fat and cholesterol have become in our culture.

But the reality is there could actually be a serious negative side effect to eating egg whites. "Egg whites contain an antinutrient called avidin, which binds biotin and prevents its absorption," nutrition scientist Dr. Chris Masterjohn told me. "In fact, a daily diet that includes 5 percent egg whites has been shown to cause birth defects in animal studies. There's evidence in humans that women who are pregnant become marginally biotin-deficient because of the stress of pregnancy. This might be a causal factor in birth defects in humans."

In Dr. Masterjohn's opinion, eating just egg whites is "probably always a bad idea," but it is especially harmful to "women of childbearing age, since they tend to be the most fearful of consuming eggs, fat, cholesterol, and red meat."

Another one of our featured experts in this book is MIT nutritional research scientist Stephanie Seneff, and she is a big advocate of animal-based foods. In fact, since saturated fats contain a key amino acid, she believes that eliminating them can cause serious health problems. "The heart, the brain, and the liver all store taurine, which is the only sulfated amino acid," said Seneff. "And taurine is only found in animal products. So if you're a vegetarian, you're getting zero taurine in your diet."

Egg yolks from pastured chickens and fresh fish already deliver large amounts of crucial omega-3 fatty acids, but they also provide all the taurine your body needs to thrive. So people eating low-fat, vegetarian diets are missing out on some of the healthiest foods you could possibly be eating for optimal heart health. "We should be eating a lot of cholesterol-containing foods," said Seneff. "I don't see how nutritionists could ever think that promoting eggs whites alone is a good idea."

As I said before, if a plant-based diet is working for you, then go for it. But if you are unsatisfied with the results you're getting from following a low-fat, vegetarian eating regimen, why not test a real foods–based, high-fat, moderate-protein, low-carb diet for thirty days to see how you do? What do you have to lose?

In the next chapter, we'll take a look at how your doctor interprets your cholesterol test results and why that may not necessarily be the best measuring stick for heart-health risk.

DOCTOR'S NOTE FROM DR. ERIC WESTMAN: I think some people can be healthy eating a low-fat diet, but the health of others can be worsened. It is definitely not the one-size-fits-all solution to preventing heart disease and diabetes that it has been touted to be.

KEY CHOLESTEROL CLARITY CONCEPTS

→ **A heart-healthy diet is often assumed to be a low-fat, vegetarian one.**

→ **When the focus is on LDL cholesterol, cutting fat and cholesterol is logical.**

→ **If you follow a low-fat, vegetarian eating regimen and are healthy, then keep doing it.**

→ **When you cut fat out of your diet, you generally replace it with more carbohydrates.**

→ **High-carb, low-fat diets increase triglycerides, lower HDL, and raise Small LDL-P.**

→ **Dr. Dean Ornish credits his low-fat diet with improving heart health.**

→ **Dr. Ornish's regimen did not prevent the patients in his study from experiencing cardiovascular events.**

→ **Dr. Ornish's study never isolated diet alone.**

→ **Lifestyle changes with the proper diet plan are essential to heart health.**

→ **Limiting egg consumption to whites only poses health problems.**

→ **Eschewing animal-based foods robs the heart, brain, and liver of vital nutrients.**

Chapter 18

How Your Doctor (Mis)Interprets Your Cholesterol Test Results

MOMENT OF CLARITY: "Somebody discovered how to measure cholesterol. And as is true in so many fields, if you can measure it, then you can do something about it."

— Dr. Dwight Lundell

MOMENT OF CLARITY: "The focus of cholesterol treatment by most of mainstream medicine has been looking at a standard lipid panel. When there are elevations in LDL and total cholesterol, that is assumed to be an indicator of an increased risk of cardiovascular disease. But that doesn't entirely capture the picture because of the research we have seen on the particle size and the various subclasses of LDL cholesterol. There's a body of evidence that has emerged showing that small, dense LDL is more strongly associated with cardiovascular disease risk than the larger, more buoyant particles. There's more to the story than just LDL cholesterol and total cholesterol. By using more sensitive testing technology and assessment strategies, we can develop more appropriate treatment for each individual."

— Dr. Patty Siri-Tarino

When you visit your primary care physician and get your cholesterol checked, you probably assume your doctor is employing some fancy-schmancy, sophisticated, modern-day methodology. In reality, though, the process is painfully primitive and simplistic—arguably the most unscientific part of today's typical medical practice.

Here are the likely recommendations you will get from your doctor if your cholesterol test reveals that you have a total cholesterol reading over 200 or an LDL-C over 100:

▶ Eat a "healthy diet," which is defined as reducing the amount of saturated fat and cholesterol you are consuming, while eating more fish; lots of fruits and vegetables; as well as plenty of "healthy," fiber-filled whole grains. In addition, opt for low-fat alternatives, like margarine and fat-free dairy, and reduce your consumption of red meat, eggs, full-fat cheese, and sodium.

▶ Take a cholesterol-lowering medication, like a statin drug, which will quickly lower your cholesterol. If you cannot tolerate these pharmaceutical drugs, then take niacin or eat fortified foods, such as margarine, orange juice, and rice milk.

▶ Exercise at least thirty minutes a day to raise your HDL and lower your triglycerides.

MOMENT OF CLARITY: "The truth about cholesterol is out there. What people need to understand is that the media has put forth this idea that cholesterol is going to hurt them in some way. Ironically, cholesterol is actually very healthy for you and you need it, for example, to construct hormones, including testosterone and estrogen, as well as vitamin D. "Cholesterol is also a vulnerable molecule that can deteriorate if it sits around at high levels for too long or if people have stress or consume too much sugar."

– Dr. David Diamond

As we've demonstrated many times in this book, this deeply held conventional medical wisdom is completely and utterly wrong. But the obsession with LDL and total cholesterol nearly demands that doctors behave this way. I was subjected to all the usual misinformation back in 2005, when my doctor discovered my total cholesterol was over 200 and my LDL-C cholesterol was over 100. It was my first visit since losing 180 pounds and getting my health back in line. I can only imagine what my doctor would say about my April 2013 test results: total cholesterol 310 and LDL-C 236. He'd be prescribing the highest statin dose possible!

Heart surgeon Dr. Dwight Lundell remembers when cholesterol became the focus of heart disease, back in the early 1970s. He had just started practicing medicine. "All of a sudden we had two emerging therapies for heart disease after having none," Dr. Lundell told me. "We had the treatment of cholesterol, which started out with niacin, clofibrate, and those kinds of things. And we had coronary bypass surgery. I've looked inside fifteen thousand coronary arteries in my career and I've looked at the junk in there. Indeed, it is yellow and ugly and it looks like our depiction of cholesterol. When surgeons started seeing that yellow, ugly stuff, everybody got excited. We had known for a long time that this plaque contained cholesterol, along with other cellular debris. But this is when the focus turned to cholesterol."

Seemingly overnight, it was assumed that if you had elevated levels of LDL and total cholesterol in your blood, they would get deposited in your coronary arteries, leading to a heart attack, heart disease, or death. Nobody challenged the theory at the time, but, even more amazingly, few have challenged it ever since despite plenty of scientific and clinical evidence to the contrary. Yet we are seeing cracks in the walls of this monolithic thinking beginning to appear.

MOMENT OF CLARITY: "There's no point in looking at the LDL cholesterol at all because it is merely calculated based on a formula and not measured directly. There's some evidence that the formula applies to some people and not to others, particularly with people who have certain variations in their triglyceride levels. If you just look at the total–to–HDL cholesterol ratio, you get rid of that problem entirely. When you look at LDL cholesterol itself, it's merely confusing the picture."

– Dr. Chris Masterjohn

The Beginning of a Cholesterol Revolution

Frustration is building over the outdated theory that LDL cholesterol is the primary target for determining heart health treatment. In an "Editor's Perspective," published in the April 19, 2012 issue of the scientific journal *Circulation: Cardiovascular Quality and Outcomes* (a subsidiary of the prestigious *Journal of the American Heart Association*), a pair of physicians named Dr. Rodney Hayward and Dr. Harlan Krumholz expressed their concern over targeting even lower levels of low-density lipoprotein (LDL) cholesterol.

They argued that focusing exclusively on LDL has never been properly researched or vetted for effectiveness or safety and that a "more tailored treatment approach," for each patient, based on that patient's specific needs, is sorely needed. Don't be surprised if you begin to hear more of this kind of talk. As Napa, California–based family physician Dr. Cate Shanahan, one of the featured experts in this book, pointed out to me, "For both LDL and total cholesterol, we have little to no data really to tell us what they mean as individual risk factors. I tell my patients that the total cholesterol is completely meaningless because it's composed partly of a number we want to be high—HDL. And it's not very reflective of another number that's very important, and that's triglycerides."

MOMENT OF CLARITY: "There are a lot of confounding variables with these lipid markers that might make it next to impossible to ever find real answers."

— Dr. Rocky Patel

Dr. Shanahan shared an analogy that perfectly illustrates the absurdity of treating patients based on their total cholesterol alone. "It would be as if you called me up one day and said, 'I'm five-foot-seven,' and I responded, 'You're taller than all my other patients, so you've got to lose weight!' You would probably respond, 'What? You don't even know how much I weigh!' It's the same kind of thing when you rely on total cholesterol to tell you that you have a problem."

It's been stated already throughout this book, but something Dr. Shanahan said reinforces the message being communicated even more.

"Just as many people with what is considered good, healthy levels of total cholesterol (below 200) have heart attacks as those with supposedly bad levels. They're almost completely identical. So how can we say total cholesterol is meaningful?"

DOCTOR'S NOTE FROM DR. ERIC WESTMAN: Even if there were "good" cholesterol and "bad" cholesterol, using the total cholesterol for a risk assessment would be useless.

What exactly does Dr. Shanahan tell her patients regarding cholesterol? "I openly tell them that cholesterol reference ranges are behind the times. And I can back that up with more recent scientific data."

Not surprisingly, she said, this is "shocking" information to people who have become "confused" by the well-oiled cholesterol-health-hypothesis machine. "I convince my patients by telling them that the laboratories are not up-to-date, and new information is around the corner; it will manifest soon. And that's totally true."

As we've also pointed out already, the numbers currently considered ideal are completely arbitrary anyway. "Just because it's on a piece of paper and came out of a machine doesn't mean some guy knows all the answers about your health," Dr. Shanahan said. "It's time to pull back the curtain on the Wizard of Oz." And that includes the more advanced tests measuring subfractions of LDL particles, which Dr. Shanahan considers a more expensive extension of the standard cholesterol testing that already exists. "Ultimately, it's just somebody's idea. They take something out of you and then they tell you what it means. It's that mentality that we're locked into—a magic act, like pulling a rabbit out of the hat. It's fakery and that's what people are paying for."

Why Physicians Ignore the Rest of Your Cholesterol Panel

So what about all the other numbers—HDL, triglycerides, and all the rest—on your cholesterol test results? Do they mean absolutely nothing? Do total and LDL cholesterol trump everything else as independent risk factors in heart health? These are the questions that medical doctors *should* be asking.

Dr. Ken Sikaris, one of the featured experts in this book from Melbourne, Australia, is one of the people who is doing just that. He has watched the cholesterol story develop over the last forty years. "The focus was put on LDL and seen to be the atherogenic particle in the 1970s," Dr. Sikaris told me. "But in the 1980s, the focus shifted to people with diabetes, who didn't necessarily have a high LDL or total cholesterol level, but clearly had an increased cardiovascular risk. That's when people started becoming interested in the properties of LDL and whether there were certain kinds that were more atherogenic than others."

That's precisely when the LDL and total cholesterol theory should have bit the dust, when the central focus of cardiovascular treatment shifted. But even as the technology progressed into the next decade, and it became possible to examine particle size difference in LDL cholesterol, the old hypothesis stuck. And, sadly, it still does to this day.

"In the '90s, we discovered that there were size differences in the LDL," Dr. Sikaris continued. "So the concept of the small, dense form of LDL showed up in a variety of disease groups and was linked to an increased risk of cardiovascular disease. That's when researchers started investigating why we have this small, dense LDL and where it came from. People with stress, obesity, and diabetes all seemed to have this small form of LDL, which was highly atherogenic. The theory that we still have today is that macrophages and the scavengers are the primary mechanism of atherosclerosis. The focus was on what would alter the LDL particle, oxidation, and glycation."

Unfortunately, that shift in focus has never translated into treatment; it remains almost entirely in the research realm. Featured expert and cardiac surgeon Dr. Donald Miller is convinced that there are powerful interests at work keeping the truth about cholesterol buried. "Here's what happened with the proponents of the cholesterol campaign, which includes the pharmaceutical industry, government agencies, the FDA, the NIH, and the major medical associations: They misled doctors," he explained. "They've convinced doctors that the cause of coronary disease is elevated cholesterol, brought on by consuming saturated fat. Thus, the way to prevent heart disease is to simply lower the cholesterol. Anything that contradicts with that is virtually ignored. There have been several books written detailing the problem with this belief about cholesterol, but people aren't paying attention to them."

Yes, it has been years since newer technology and advances in science have proven the old hypothesis wrong, and yet it continues to be heralded as the gospel truth. At this point, said Dr. Miller, "It's almost a religion."

There was a time even Dr. Miller accepted the cholesterol theory. His opinion didn't change until he started doing his own research. In fact, he was "shocked" by how little evidence there was for a hypothesis the medical industry deems irrefutable. These days he is presenting lectures and posting YouTube videos sharing the truth. Nevertheless, his fellow doctors don't want to hear what he has to say. "I'm alone here on an island with colleagues who refuse to talk to me about it," said Dr. Miller. "They think I'm just an eccentric old surgeon."

He revealed that he hasn't measured his cholesterol in four decades and that's what he advises professionally. "I tell people to quit getting your cholesterol measured—just stop doing it," Dr. Miller said. "All it does is raise red flags that have no basis in solid evidence. The sad thing about this is that you've got all these doctors who have been indoctrinated with the cholesterol message and they are completely clueless about the role nutrition plays. They're not taught anything about nutrition."

If you learn nothing else from reading *Cholesterol Clarity*, we hope you realize the vital role that what you are eating plays on the cholesterol levels in your blood. Nutrition is integral to optimal health and self-care, and yet the majority of doctors get next to zero education in this area. That, to me, is criminal considering all the dietary advice being given to patients by medical doctors untrained in nutrition.

Overcoming Years of Dietary Dogma Will Be Very Difficult

The powerful negative images people have about cholesterol and saturated fat will be, according to Dr. Malcolm Kendrick, "very difficult to dislodge. I don't know what you can do about people thinking that fat and cholesterol are clogging their arteries. They see these pictures of fat and then they see pictures of pipes with fat stuck in them and they're told that is what is happening to their arteries. It's a very simple story that just happens to be completely wrong. But what do you replace it with?"

Dr. Kendrick worries that changing the mind-set of people—from describing fat and cholesterol as inherently evil to now actually labeling these as healthy—might be next to impossible. "People just wouldn't believe it because you're trying to change a very powerful image in their minds," Dr. Kendrick said. "They just don't want to change. When something is bad, it's bad; when something is good, it's good. Changing something from good to bad or bad to good in the emotional context of people's brains is very difficult."

I understand Dr. Kendrick's concern, but I have hope moving forward, based on my own experience and the experiences of others, including British medical doctor and nutritional health author Dr. John Briffa. "For me, hope comes from the fact that there's a large number of 'swing voters' regarding cholesterol; people who are open to new ideas about the role of cholesterol in health and how best to look after our heart and wider health," Dr. Briffa told me. "Increasingly, there is recognition that bringing cholesterol levels down is not broadly beneficial for health. We know that because almost all the cholesterol-modifying strategies that have been tried have not been found to reduce overall risk of death, even in people with high risk of cardiovascular disease. In fact, sometimes, specific drugs have been found to have adverse effects on health and even kill people."

A New Way to Assess Cardiovascular Risk

Doubt is a great thing: It opens the door, even if it's by only a crack, to alternative theories. Once you've allowed more information in, you can begin to make informed decisions about your own health.

The first thing you should be questioning, according to Dr. Kendrick, is the current method for assessing cardiovascular health—the one used in virtually every doctor's office around the world. "The power of the measurement itself is something you're fighting against with cholesterol testing," he said. "That's one of the reasons why I am measuring in a different way now—a way that reveals a true measurement, one that might mean something. I think this is quite important."

The allure of going to your doctor's office and seeing a number you can improve is understandable and that appeal is universal. Doctors like it and so do their patients. Who doesn't like quantifiable change? But what if the numbers don't mean anything? Shouldn't you find numbers that *do* mean something? That's why Dr. Kendrick now uses a different set of measurements, one that gives a more well-rounded and accurate reading on the current state of the patients' health and metabolism with meaningful recommendations they can act upon. "These tools are used to determine whether my patient is burning fat or sugar," Dr. Kendrick explained. "That's why we are directing people toward higher-fat diets. You can't lose weight if you are burning sugar, and we show them, through measurements on a machine, that if you reduce your carbohydrate intake and increase your fat intake, your ability to lose weight dramatically improves. We're actually developing evidence now to show this to patients."

This is the kind of "evidence" doctors and patients need. Dr. Fred Pescatore agrees with Dr. Kendrick; he, too, doesn't "get concerned much with cholesterol levels. Your own body makes 80 percent of the cholesterol you have. So if the body is making cholesterol, there's a reason for it to be there. To think that we need to reduce it to levels that are suboptimal is kind of silly."

Dr. Pescatore said the only merit to checking cholesterol is that it "can be a marker for something else going on in the body." But worrying about cholesterol itself as a causal factor in heart disease is pure folly. "Cholesterol is not what kills you," he explained. "Cholesterol increases in response to oxidative stress. If you get rid of the oxidative stress, then cholesterol levels will go down automatically."

And what about the unfounded fear that higher cholesterol levels lead to the rapid development of clogged arteries? "Cholesterol in the blood doesn't mean you're going to have plaque formation that's going to make you die," Dr. Pescatore noted. "It's there to help and heal whatever damage is being done. It gets a bad rap."

While he does test for cholesterol levels in patients who request them, "I never do anything about it. You need to see the whole picture and not focus too much on any one marker," Dr. Pescatore explained. "Your body is not just your cholesterol number. Your body and your cardiovascular health include an entire spectrum of things that need to be looked at."

MOMENT OF CLARITY: "It was decided to settle on cholesterol as the indirect means for quantifying these particles. That's when they started to measure the cholesterol, the various fractions in the blood—low-density lipoprotein (LDL) cholesterol, high-density lipoprotein (HDL) cholesterol, total cholesterol, very low-density lipoprotein (VLDL) cholesterol. Somehow in all of this, cholesterol got misconstrued as being the cause of heart disease when all it was really ever meant to be was the yardstick. It was simply a measuring stick for these particles. Fast-forward forty years: We now treat cholesterol—a mere measuring stick of potential heart disease risk and not necessarily the causal factor."

– Dr. William Davis

In the next chapter we'll take a look at the numbers on your basic cholesterol test and help you to understand what they mean in terms of your own personal health. If you have cholesterol numbers outside the normal or supposedly healthy range, then this is the section of the book you've been waiting for. Even if I've managed to convince you that cholesterol numbers don't really matter, it's worth understanding the various ranges you should be shooting for and what you can do to reach those levels if there are any lingering doubts.

DOCTOR'S NOTE FROM DR. ERIC WESTMAN: We have learned a tremendous amount about the effect of diet on blood cholesterol over the last ten to fifteen years. If a recommendation was created before that time and hasn't changed, then it can't be up-to-date. Most of what was predicted about what would happen with the low-carb, high-fat diet didn't come true when the studies were finally done.

KEY CHOLESTEROL CLARITY CONCEPTS

→ **Cholesterol science has changed over the years, but the treatment has not.**

→ **Many medical professionals are beginning to doubt cholesterol's role in heart disease.**

→ **People are shocked to find out that LDL and total cholesterol are meaningless numbers.**

→ **Cholesterol testing is just a diagnostic tool; it is not intended for doctors to treat anything.**

→ **The shift in cholesterol technology happened on the research—not the clinical—level.**

→ **The cholesterol theory of heart disease is widely believed, like a religion.**

→ **Stop measuring your cholesterol and avoid the fears associated with it.**

→ **Changing the negative images about cholesterol is very difficult.**

→ **New tools are being developed for patients to track their health progress.**

→ **The only value in checking cholesterol is in helping to identify other health issues.**

→ **Cholesterol in the blood does not mean it will become deposited in arteries.**

Chapter 19

What Your Basic Cholesterol Test Results Mean

MOMENT OF CLARITY: "I actually think you can do fine without advanced testing. It may be just an expensive way to get information that we already get on the standard cholesterol testing we've been running for thirty years."

— Dr. Jeffry Gerber

Hopefully, you now understand that elevated cholesterol is neither a disease nor a definite causal factor in heart disease. (This is a recording!) But you might still be wondering what your cholesterol test results *do* tell you. Can they be an indication of problems? Yes! And are there ideal ranges you should shoot for? Yes!

Most of you have probably had your basic cholesterol numbers run by your doctor—your total cholesterol, LDL-C, HDL-C, VLDL-C, and triglycerides. We'll zero in on each of these in this chapter. We'll also take a look what it means to have a number that is marked in red or labeled as "high," "low," or "out of range," and tell you what mainstream medical health sources say about those numbers. Finally, we'll provide you with the optimal levels you should be striving for. Here's where the rubber meets the road with your cholesterol numbers, so go grab your test results so you can see how you are doing! It's time to bring crystal-clear clarity to the cholesterol confusion.

MOMENT OF CLARITY: "Using lipid concentrations from the standard lipid profile is the most accurate way of assessing cardiovascular risk. It's better than nothing—that's for sure."

— Dr. Thomas Dayspring

Total Cholesterol

What is it?

In a nutshell, your total cholesterol is the combined total of LDL-C, HDL-C, and VLDL-C. Honestly, this number doesn't tell you a whole lot about your health. Someone once told me that knowing your total cholesterol is the same as knowing that the total score at the end of a baseball game is 25. You don't know how each player did or how intense the competition was. The game could have been a nail-biter—a 13–12 game—or maybe a complete blowout of 24–1. In the same way, you can't know your real health story by looking at just one marker like total cholesterol.

What do mainstream health experts consider the ideal range?

Desirable: below 200 mg/dL
Borderline: 200–239 mg/dL
High: 240+ mg/dL
Source: MayoClinic.com

What are optimal levels for good health?

Conventional wisdom calls for keeping total cholesterol below 200, but there's no scientific basis for this; it's a totally arbitrary level. It also isn't a reliable marker for determining your risk of heart disease. So attempting to lower the total number makes no sense at all. More important than the totality of the number is what the number is composed of.

New thinking based on normal cholesterol levels in traditional cultures free from heart disease proposes the following: For women, a total cholesterol of 250 mg/dL or below is considered normal, and for men a total of 220 mg/dL or below is viewed as normal. Levels above these cutoff points are not necessarily an indication of a need for pharmaceutical therapy, but rather an indication that you should look into other factors regarding your overall health.

Can you lower total cholesterol naturally?

Since total cholesterol doesn't really mean anything in terms of cardiovascular health, trying to lower it is pretty much a useless endeavor. As we've discussed, cholesterol is in your body for a reason and unnecessarily manipulating it nutritionally or with a prescription drug may be more harmful than helpful. Rather than worrying about the total cholesterol number, talk with your doctor about what might be the underlying cause of your elevated total cholesterol, including the possibilities discussed in chapters 14 and 15.

LDL-C

MOMENT OF CLARITY: "LDL is extremely important for your immunity. If you've got too little, then you may not mount an appropriate immune response to infections. But if you have too much, then you might have an overactive immune response, which could lead to various problems, such as excess inflammation."

– Paul Jaminet

What is it?

Commonly referred to as "bad" cholesterol, LDL stands for "low-density lipoprotein" and it enables fat molecules to be transported through the bloodstream. While LDL is typically viewed by many physicians as just one number, it's actually a combination of two primary types: the large, fluffy Pattern A and the small, dense Pattern B. We'll discuss these concepts in greater detail in the next chapter.

The LDL-C on your basic cholesterol test result is a calculated number based on estimates using the Friedewald equation, which is formulated by taking your total cholesterol value and subtracting your HDL and then subtracting your triglycerides divided by 5. That is more information than you probably want to know, but stick with me because this is important to understand. The Friedewald equation has known discrepancies that make this calculated LDL-C number extremely unreliable. So why is it used? It is much more affordable than determining direct measurements of LDL cholesterol. But, again, the results are significantly flawed and virtually meaningless.

Ideal LDL-C ranges, according to mainstream health experts:

People at very high risk of heart disease: below 70 mg/dL
People at high risk of heart disease: below 100 mg/dL
Near ideal: 100–129 mg/dL
Borderline high risk of heart disease: 130–159 mg/dL
High: 160–189 mg/dL
Very high: 190+ mg/dL
Source: MayoClinic.com

What are optimal levels for health?

Mainstream medical experts advise those at "very high risk of heart dis-ease" to keep their LDL-C number below 100, or even below 70. But, again, I must ask why, especially when 50 percent of heart attack victims have "normal" LDL cholesterol levels? If LDL-C actually indicated heart health, lowering it to the above levels, by whatever means necessary, would make sense. But that's not the case.

Additionally, as we have already discussed, LDL isn't just one number. A level of 100 doesn't, for example, tell you a whole lot about LDL particles; it's their size and number that are of critical importance. Dr. Paul Jaminet believes the ideal level for LDL cholesterol is 130 mg/dL—a bit higher than what mainstream medicine says is healthy. Generally speaking, you don't want too little LDL cholesterol or too much; the latter can lead to an increase in inflammation, which shows up in your C-reactive protein levels (another important health marker discussed in the next chapter). So your LDL-C level is much like total cholesterol: As a singular marker, it doesn't tell you much about your health.

Can you lower LDL-C naturally?

As with total cholesterol, the results are flawed and virtually meaningless, so don't worry about lowering it.

HDL-C

What is it?

HDL (high-density lipoprotein) is the smallest of the lipoprotein particles. It enables the transportation of triglycerides through the bloodstream; in healthy people, about 30 percent of fat in the blood is carried by HDL. It also utilizes and excretes LDL from the body by delivering it to the liver. In essence, HDL acts as a cleanser of the endothelium, or the inner linings of the blood vessels. When your endothelium gets damaged, that can lead to atherosclerosis, which causes a heart attack or stroke. This is why HDL is often referred to as the "good" cholesterol. An increased level of HDL-C is thus protective against cardiovascular disease, while lower levels of HDL-C tend to raise your risk of heart disease. Men tend to have lower HDL than women do.

What range do mainstream health experts want you to have?

Poor: below 40 mg/dL (men) or below 50 mg/dL (women)

Better: 40–49 mg/dL (men) or 50–59 mg/dL (women)

Best: 60+ mg/dL

Source: MayoClinic.com

What are the optimal levels for good health?

HDL has been all but ignored by mainstream medicine, which focuses almost exclusively on LDL and total cholesterol. And yet it can be argued that this number (along with triglycerides) is the best predictor of heart disease risk. To derive the biggest benefits for your cardiovascular health, you want your HDL cholesterol at 70 mg/dL or higher, which is more than what mainstream experts recommend. Anything below 50 should be cause for concern.

Can you raise HDL naturally?

If you love consuming animal fats but have cut back to keep your cholesterol numbers down, take heart: One of the best ways to raise your HDL cholesterol is to consume more dietary fats, including healthy saturated fats, such as coconut oil, butter, cream, full-fat meats, and dairy, as well as monounsaturated fats like avocados and olive oil. Sounds too good to be true, right? But consuming a high-fat diet provides your body with the raw materials for making HDL cholesterol. Additionally, HDL production responds to regular exercise, reducing alcohol consumption, and (if you're up for it) periodic, intermittent fasting of sixteen hours at a time.

VLDL-C

MOMENT OF CLARITY: "Showing the VLDL improvements when you reduce your carbohydrate intake is an important number; it demonstrates to patients how they are improving."

— Dr. Malcolm Kendrick

MOMENT OF CLARITY: "Lipidologists realize the connection between blood sugar control, cholesterol, and heart disease. Or at least they should. When you are in a state of carbohydrate excess, the very first sign that I see that on a cholesterol lab panel is a high VLDL-3. Then, over time, triglycerides rapidly increasing would be the second sign that a person is eating too many carbs. I see a lot of patients with insulin resistance with 'normal' triglyceride levels around 150, but their VLDL-3 is high. So if patients with these kinds of numbers tell me they are following the low-carb diet, I know they're not because the VLDL-3 levels would have come down."

– Dr. Rocky Patel

What is it?

VLDL is an acronym for "very low-density lipoproteins." These are made in the liver and carry triglycerides and other fats in the blood throughout the body. VLDL is widely considered bad cholesterol because higher levels indicate an increase in the blood concentration of triglycerides. You can usually calculate your VLDL-C by dividing your triglycerides by 5.

Ideal VLDL range, according to mainstream health experts

Normal: between 2 and 30 mg/dL

Source: National Institutes of Health

What are the optimal levels for good health?

The "normal" recommended range for VLDL-C is so wide as to be rendered meaningless. There's a big difference between having a VLDL of 2 or a VLDL of 30. In general, the lower you can make your VLDL-C, the better off your heart health will be. Aim for between 10 and 14 mg/dL VLDL.

Can you lower VLDL naturally?

Preventing or reducing insulin resistance is essential to keeping VLDL at optimal levels. The fastest way to do that is to eliminate or dramatically reduce consumption of carbohydrates, and particularly refined carbs, like white bread, white rice, pasta, and junk foods, as well as sugar, wheat, potatoes, brown rice, and starchy vegetables.

Triglycerides

MOMENT OF CLARITY: "Raised triglycerides or VLDL is a result of the body not dealing with sugar and fat properly. Once you develop insulin resistance, all the other aspects of your health start to go awry. Asian-Indians, as we call them in the UK, are often not obese and have low LDL cholesterol, but these guys are developing central obesity and insulin resistance and they just die really young."

— Dr. Malcolm Kendrick

What are they?

Triglycerides are fats composed of three fatty acids. Their very important job is to transfer the fat and blood glucose—the energy your body needs— from the liver. When they are elevated, it means that your risk of heart disease increases. In fact, your triglyceride level inversely correlates with a low level of HDL cholesterol; when triglycerides are high, HDL cholesterol tends to be low. The more triglycerides you have in your blood, the greater your chance of developing atherosclerosis.

Ideal triglyceride range, according to mainstream health experts:

Desirable: below 150 mg/dL
Borderline high: 150–199 mg/dL
High: 200–499 mg/dL
Very high: 500+ mg/dL
Source: MayoClinic.com

What are optimal levels for good health?

Here's where reality veers dramatically from conventional wisdom: The "desirable" number promoted by mainstream health experts is ridiculously high. Instead of 150 mg/dL, you should be aiming for 100 mg/dL or *less*. In fact, we suggest 70mg/dL as the optimal range for healthy triglyceride levels.

Can you lower triglycerides naturally?

Sorry if I'm beginning to sound like a broken record, but I can't resist the song: Decrease your carbohydrates! Do this and your triglycerides will drop like a rock. My wife Christine is the perfect example of this. She had triglycerides pushing 300 mg/dL in 2008 and, in just six weeks, got that number down to 130 by eating a low-carb diet and taking a cod liver oil supplement. When she kicked her M&Ms and Skittles habit, her triglycerides dropped even further, to an amazing 43 mg/dL.

MOMENT OF CLARITY: "As triglycerides go up, the HDL goes down and the VLDL remains elevated."

– Dr. Rocky Patel

In the next chapter, we'll take a look at some of the more advanced cholesterol tests. Some would argue that you don't really need any of these fancy tests, but I do find them helpful for those who are concerned about their health. These tests provide a reliable snapshot of both cardiovascular and overall health.

MOMENT OF CLARITY: "The level of triglycerides that predicts small, dense LDL is much lower than what is considered the normal range. It's better to have below-average levels than above-average, but it's even better to be below the lower twenty-fifth percentile than the upper twenty-fifth percentile. It's a continuum: The lower you get, the less your risk. Nobody has ever looked for what a healthy level is. It's all about the relative risk of heart disease. But some are pushing for the absolute risk of heart disease."

– Dr. Ken Sikaris

DOCTOR'S NOTE FROM DR. ERIC WESTMAN: In very rare circumstances, the blood cholesterol or triglycerides can build up under the skin or in the tissue. These buildups may represent rare familial problems that can lead to early heart disease, and treatment may lower this risk. If you see these fatty accumulations, then definitely get your blood cholesterol levels checked.

KEY CHOLESTEROL CLARITY CONCEPTS

→ **Most doctors run a basic cholesterol panel: total, LDL, HDL, VLDL and triglycerides.**

→ **Total cholesterol is virtually meaningless because it doesn't reveal the makeup of the cholesterol.**

→ **The LDL-C level is also virtually meaningless, since it's the particles that matter.**

→ **HDL and triglycerides are the two most important numbers on your test results.**

→ **VLDL is an outstanding proxy for triglycerides and should be as low as possible.**

→ **Eating a high-fat, low-carb diet will dramatically improve HDL and triglycerides.**

Chapter 20
Eight Advanced Health Markers You Should Consider

MOMENT OF CLARITY: "Progressive lipidologists are more concerned with LDL particles, ApoB, and the more modern technology for measuring lipoproteins. But this twenty-first-century science is deemed much too complicated and confusing by the authorities looking at cholesterol. The catch is that this newer information has been sealed off from the general public as well as the very people who are producing the latest cholesterol guidelines."

— **Gary Taubes**

We already talked about the various companies offering advanced cholesterol testing. Now we'll get into the more sophisticated measurements these companies offer—tests you should consider if you or your doctor are concerned about your basic cholesterol test numbers. Your doctor can run any of them, but so can you, via the medical testing websites cited in chapter 9.

1. Apolipoprotein B (ApoB)

MOMENT OF CLARITY: "All the evidence has shown that having a high ApoB number means you are at risk of atherosclerosis. Of course, there are exceptions to this, but how can you know if this applies to you? If you want to make the choice not to worry about ApoB, then at least have a regular CT heart calcium score. If you are a male, it should be less than 50 and for women less than 60. Also you can get a carotid IMT conducted. If that's staying good, then perhaps you're not as much at risk."

— **Dr. Thomas Dayspring**

The purpose of Apolipoprotein B, or ApoB, is to carry LDL cholesterol to the tissues. The ApoB test is only ten years old, but it's already cheap and readily available throughout the world. Higher levels of ApoB are an indicator of heart disease risk, but because the test is relatively new there isn't enough data to make it as ubiquitous as LDL-C. That doesn't stop Denver family physician Dr. Jeffry Gerber from using it as a tool to measure risk. "I like ApoB testing. There are two school buses that carry cholesterol. The bad school bus is the ApoB school bus. ApoB carries cholesterol in a bad way because it carries passengers like chylomicrons, IDL, VLDL, LDL and Lp(a). These are all the bad particles that comprise the ApoB number. I like to focus on ApoB because it really provides us with a snapshot of all the supposedly harmful lipoprotein particles. ApoB gives you a more accurate measurement of the unhealthy particles."

2. LDL-P

MOMENT OF CLARITY: "Certainly, right now, particle numbers of certain lipoproteins are much better indicators of who gets atherosclerosis or not than a standard cholesterol measurement."

— Dr. Thomas Dayspring

I would venture to guess that most people reading this book have never heard of LDL-P. LDL has traditionally been measured on most cholesterol tests as LDL-C. But now we have more sophisticated ways to measure LDL—ways that can actually look at the number and size of the LDL particles you have in your blood. (The *P* in LDL-P stands for the total particles it contains.) Even Dr. Mehmet Oz, host of the popular television health program *The Dr. Oz Show*, has emphasized the importance of the Particle Size Test in determining heart health.

The best test for measuring LDL particles is the NMR Lipoprofile test from Liposcience in Raleigh, North Carolina. *NMR* is the acronym for "nuclear magnetic resonance" and it is the best commercial lab test using this state-of-the-art technology to determine the nature of your LDL particles—whether they are mostly the large, fluffy Pattern A kind (the good ones) or the small, dense Pattern B type (the bad ones). Your LDL-P number is far more relevant to heart health than your LDL-C will ever be.

There is still debate among lipidologists over whether it is the total number of LDL particles or the size of the particles that matters most. (We'll take a closer look at the size issue in the next marker.) The common use of NMR technology in medical practice is still very new, but right now Liposcience recommends LDL-P below 1,000 nmol/L as the optimal level. As we discussed in chapter 14, LDL-P can tend to go up much higher than this in people consuming a low-carb, high-fat diet and there is no research into what this means yet.

MOMENT OF CLARITY: "I'm a centrist. I'm in the middle of all this debate over LDL-P versus the size of the LDL particles. Certainly we know that Small LDL-P is significantly more atherogenic, but that might not be the complete picture. But elevated Small LDL-P is probably a surrogate for insulin resistance. However, if you're not looking for insulin resistance or taking into account inflammation, then you have to look at everything."

– Dr. Rocky Patel

3. Small LDL-P

MOMENT OF CLARITY: "Small LDL-P is another marker that invariably improves for any patient who eats a low-carb diet. It's the great trifecta—triglycerides drop, HDL goes up, and LDL particle size increases."

– Dr. Jeffry Gerber

When you get an NMR Lipoprofile test, the results include a separate listing for Small LDL-P. This is the number of LDL particles that are classified as Pattern B—the dense and truly dangerous type that you want to avoid at all costs. Cardiologist Dr. William Davis has described Small LDL-P as "far and away the number-one cause of heart disease."

"I think both your LDL-P and Small LDL-P numbers matter, but I believe small LDL particles matter a whole bunch more," Dr. Davis told me. "We don't currently have a long-term outcome study comparing treatment methods, so it's impossible to know the best way to reduce Small LDL-P levels. That hasn't been done because there's no drug for it and nobody is willing to pay the $30 million it would take to do such a study. That's generally why the drug companies perform these studies."

This major gap in the research has not stopped medical professionals like Dr. Davis from taking steps to help their patients lower their Small LDL-P with basic nutrition. "The mix of things required to do that is very simple and it hints at most of the underlying causes of coronary disease," said Dr. Davis. "We take out all wheat and limit carbohydrates in the diet. Those are the foods that trigger the formation of small LDL particles, the most flagrant, abnormal pattern that occurs in people with coronary disease and cardiovascular risk."

Small LDL-P is also much harder to get rid of once it is in your body. "Compared to the larger particles, these are much more long-lived," Dr. Davis continued. "In other words, if I have some fatty foods and that raises my large LDL, then that persists for about twenty-four hours. But if I eat a carbohydrate-rich food like bread, and it triggers the formation of small LDL, that could stick around for at least a week, if not several weeks."

Small LDL-P is prone to a process called glycation, which makes the particles stickier than large LDL particles—a big reason why, according to Dr. Davis, these smaller, denser particles are "uncommonly long-lived and very unforgiving. Although small LDL is poorly recognized by the liver, it is wonderfully recognized by inflammatory white blood cells, like the mast cells and macrophages that live in plaque. That's why small LDL is much more likely to trigger a cascade of inflammatory events. It's got a mask on, it's got mud on its shoes, it's got a sly look on its face, and it looks like the cause for heart disease. We just don't have those outcome studies."

While the serious research into this Small LDL-P issue continues, Dr. Davis recommends that people educate themselves: "I should caution people that their doctors may say not to worry about small LDL—if they even know what that is—if their HDL is above 40. I don't know where they got that fiction from. That is complete nonsense!"

In general, having higher levels of HDL cholesterol and lower levels of triglycerides, which we discussed in the previous chapter, will tend to result in a reduced Small LDL-P number.

MOMENT OF CLARITY: "In the five to ten years that the concept of small, dense LDL went from the hypothetical to proven, we had this massive growth in obesity. So the prevalence of obesity and high triglycerides was growing as well. This made people realize that this was not just important for some patients, but even for those with the most common lipid abnormality, which we now know is an elevated triglyceride level."

— Dr. Ken Sikaris

As I mentioned earlier, there is still a fair amount of controversy over LDL particles and their significance and, particularly, the total number of particles versus particle size. Research so far has seemingly favored the total LDL particle number, but Dr. Ronald Krauss, a highly-respected cholesterol researcher and featured expert in this book, agrees with Dr. Davis that your Small LDL-P level seems to be more indicative of heart disease. "A flawed statistical analysis is what has led to the conclusion that the large LDL particles are as atherogenic as the small LDL particles," Dr. Krauss explained. "I just don't believe that's true. I think there are a number of lines of evidence that suggest that's not true."

He noted that a patient with a lot of very small LDL particles has "a different pathology" than if most of the LDL particles are large. "When I see patients who have a lot of very small LDL, their LDL-C may be totally normal but their LDL particle concentration is usually elevated.

Dr. Krauss believes, once again, that carbs are the villain in this story. "Carbohydrates drive the production of fat in the liver and visceral fat," he said. "And we think the liver fat—which is unfortunately elevated in a lot of people with metabolic syndrome—stimulates the production of VLDL, which not only gives rise to these small and very small LDL, but leads to reductions in HDL. This generates the triad of high triglycerides, increased levels of small LDL, and reduced levels of HDL cholesterol."

What leads to lower HDL cholesterol, higher VLDL, and an overabundance of Small LDL-P is increased triglycerides from carbohydrate-based foods. It's a vicious cycle that puts you on a one-way path to a bona fide heart crisis.

One of Dr. Krauss's fellow cholesterol researchers, Dr. Patty Siri-Tarino, concurs. "With Small LDL-P, you'll often see other metabolic abnormalities, including elevations in triglycerides and reductions in HDL cholesterol," Dr. Siri-Tarino said. "It's part of a pattern. And that's related to a particular metabolic pathway that we believe to be, in part, induced by a high-carbohydrate diet, insulin resistance, and obesity."

> **MOMENT OF CLARITY:** "LDL particle size matters because the large, fluffy kind are hard to oxidize because the lipoprotein is protected by a lot of fats. Fats are very light, so fat-rich LDL particles float. By contrast, proteins are denser than blood so an LDL particle that doesn't have much fat is called a small, dense LDL particle (Small LDL-P). These tend to sink and, more important, the protein is exposed and is very quick to oxidize. Having lots of small, dense LDL means you have a jumpy immune system that is very sensitive. It mounts a very strong immune response. However, if you have the fatty, fluffy kind of LDL, then you'll have a quieter immune response."
>
> – Paul Jaminet

The people at Liposcience recommend having less than 600 nmol/L of Small LDL-P. That is certainly an admirable goal, but hardly ideal if you have a recommended total LDL-P of 1,000; that would mean that over half your LDL particles are the bad kind! Small LDL-P should be closer to 20 percent or less of your total LDL particles and optimally less than 200 nmol/L.

Simply put: To minimize or prevent damage to your arterial walls, you want as few small, dense LDL particles as possible. And the best way to achieve that is by consuming fewer carbohydrates, eating more saturated fats and cholesterol in your diet, exercising, and losing weight. Sound familiar?

4. Non-HDL Cholesterol

> **MOMENT OF CLARITY:** "Why does the total–to–HDL cholesterol ratio have predictive value in cardiovascular health? My working hypothesis is that it acts as a marker for the time that the LDL particles spend in the blood. There's overwhelming evidence that if you block the metabolism of LDL cholesterol, then you increase the time it spends in the blood and increase the likelihood of it becoming oxidized. Once LDL becomes oxidized or damaged, then it becomes a problem. The other problem is that when the total–to–HDL cholesterol ratio is out of whack, it's a possible indicator of this metabolic backup. And if that metabolic backup is there, then that is what needs to be fixed. So the emphasis

isn't on lowering total cholesterol; we're increasing the HDL cholesterol and reju-
venating the metabolism of the lipids to get everything back in order."

– Dr. Chris Masterjohn

You may have seen non-HDL cholesterol pop up on your standard
cholesterol test, and I'm going to guess you had no idea what it meant. It's
important because, unlike looking at total cholesterol or LDL-C, it takes
into account your VLDL-C, and for that reason Dr. Rocky Patel considers
it invaluable: "Non-HDL is a free test since it's already on your standard
lipid panel. It's just a calculation of total cholesterol minus HDL. Most of
the labs are now reporting non-HDL. You'll catch a whole lot more people
with problems looking at non-HDL than you would just looking at LDL-C."

Dr. Patel told me that non-HDL cholesterol is also an excellent proxy for
ApoB and LDL-P, particularly for people who can't afford to test for those
things. "If you really want to go the route of testing for all these things, you
can," he said. "But I don't think you necessarily need to. If your non-HDL is
high, that means you've got a lot of lipoproteins in the system requiring you
to start doing something different."

Dr. Patel thinks non-HDL cholesterol should be included as a target in
the next ATP IV Cholesterol Guidelines, since, even more than LDL-C, it
"acts as a surrogate marker for lipoprotein counts and not just LDL concentration counts."

Dr. Krauss likes non-HDL cholesterol as well, because it is a simple test
for assessing lipid-related risk. "It is consistent with all the current guidelines and goes a long way toward helping to assess heart disease risk in the
general population," Dr. Krauss said. "Part of the reason the marketing of
non-HDL cholesterol has been a dismal failure is because it has a strange
name. It was proposed in the previous ATP Guidelines for the first time,
but it was confusing to people and it hasn't been embraced. I would suggest calling it something like 'atherogenic cholesterol.' It needs a name that
clearly says it's bad."

The ideal level of non-HDL cholesterol is still to be determined. Depending on your LDL target for your personal health situation, conventional
wisdom says to add 30 to that (because VLDL is your triglycerides divided
by 5, and a triglyceride level of 150 is deemed optimal). But, as Dr. Krauss
has pointed out, "there's no real evidence for picking a specific cutoff point
for non-HDL cholesterol."

5. Lipoprotein(a)

This is another one of those heart-health markers you probably haven't seen or heard much about. But Lipoprotein(a)—commonly referred to as Lp(a)—has been identified as a key genetic risk factor in coronary artery disease and stroke. It's made up of an LDL-like particle and is mostly predetermined by the genes you inherited from your parents. Because it is genetically based, and therefore commonly thought that you can't do much about it, many doctors ignore it. That is shortsighted, as you will discover in a moment.

There's still a lot being learned about Lp(a), but we do know that people with lower levels tend to be healthier than those with high Lp(a). The healthy ranges for Lp(a) vary widely— between 5 and 40 mg/dL. Because there are several different ways to measure it, there is no standard testing methodology that provides consistent and relevant reference ranges.

MOMENT OF CLARITY: "About 25 percent of the population have levels of Lp(a) that can put them at higher heart disease risk, so it's not rare at all."

– Dr. Ronald Krauss

Because Lp(a) is still so new and there are several ways to calculate it, there is enormous difficulty in attempting to target an optimal level. But since it doesn't appear to serve any good physiological purpose, common sense suggests that you keep it as low as possible. But the Lp(a) story is far more complicated than that.

MOMENT OF CLARITY: "Lipoprotein(a) is a blood-clotting agent, essentially a thrombus. Therefore, when you find them stuck inside artery walls, you're not actually looking at LDL, you're looking at Lp(a). People have refused to recognize that is what they are looking at."

– Dr. Malcolm Kendrick

Dr. William Davis has researched Lp(a) extensively over many years. He's made some rather keen observations about people with a strong genetic predisposition to increased levels of Lp(a).

"Do you know what I call people with Lp(a)?" he asked me. "They're perfect carnivores. In our modern-day world, Lp(a) is an extravagant cardiovascular risk. You hear about families where a guy has a heart attack at forty-two, his dad had a heart attack or bypass at forty-seven, and a woman in the family has a heart attack at age fifty-two. More often than not, that is a Lp(a)-bearing family. But let me tell you what I really think, based on my very large experience of working with people who have Lp(a). If you collected one hundred people with high Lp(a) and just watched them, you'll notice several curious things. They're all very athletic, with 80 percent of them being triathletes, marathon runners, or long-distance exercisers. It's going to sound crazy, but the guys are very good at math. I recognize an Lp(a) guy when he comes into my office with his cholesterol values, blood sugars, blood pressures, and other health numbers for the last ten years sketched out in an Excel spreadsheet and graphed for you. I know these guys have Lp(a) because they have uncommon gifts for math. They're smart.

"They also have an increased tolerance for dehydration as well as starvation. Plus, they have a heightened immunity to tropical infections. In other words, they are the ultimate example of this notion of a 'thrifty gene' because they are incredibly good survivors. They're the people who can outwit predators and other humans in the wild because they can spear their prey to injure it and chase it down for five hours without stopping to drink or eat.

"As I've described them, they are perfect carnivores. Because Lp(a) appeared in primates only a few million years ago as a rare mutation, today it is in 11 percent of humans. In other words, it's been enriched. Genes don't become enriched because they are bad, but because they're good."

Fascinating! Dr. Davis says high Lp(a) in the days of our early ancestors was "a gift of nature that gave people an incredible survival advantage." So if it's a gift that allowed our hunter-gather forebears to survive in the worst of circumstances, why is Lp(a) such a strong risk factor for heart disease in modern-day society?

"Over and over again, I come to the same conclusion: It's a lack of fats and overexposure to grains and sugars," Dr. Davis explained. "When Lp(a) people—more so than anyone else—cut their fat and eat more whole grains and sugar, they will display these metabolic distortions, including explosive degrees of small LDL particles, high triglycerides, and high blood sugar levels sufficient to be a diabetic. I'm talking about a six-foot-four-inch-tall, 140-pound guy who has 9 percent body fat, runs eight miles a day, and has diabetic blood sugars. So we're talking about a potential for diabetes that is out of proportion—far more than other people."

MOMENT OF CLARITY: "We're finding that people with gluten and grain sensitivity tend to have a predictable increase in inflammatory markers, as well as LDL particle issues. If you go down the low-carb route, you'll kill two birds with one stone with that. Gluten-related abnormalities are probably way bigger an issue than we ever realized before."

– Dr. Thomas Dayspring

For years the assumption has been that people with high Lp(a) had drawn the short stick in life's lottery. All they could do was take niacin or statin drugs. Dr. Davis made the critical connection between these people and the "carnivorous, high-fat lifestyle of our ancestors, where the fat of animals was eaten as well as the meat." His patients with high Lp(a) all had this genetic predisposition to survive and thrive in common.

"I have now dropped Lp(a) to zero from high levels in forty people," Dr. Davis revealed. "This isn't proof of anything, but it's very interesting. I can tell you, I've never seen Lp(a) drop to zero before. But we're doing it."

In addition to encouraging his patients to eat lots of fatty meats, Dr. Davis recommends omega-3 fats from fish and the brains of humanely raised animals. If these options are not available or are undesirable, he recommends taking a high-dose fish oil supplement. "I use 6,000 mg EPA/DHA from fish oil and that helps lower Lp(a)," Dr. Davis said. "It takes two to three years to bring these levels down; it doesn't happen overnight. But we've seen that number ratchet down further and further."

MOMENT OF CLARITY: "There is a distinction between absolute risk and relative risk. For example, if patients have Lp(a) that's through the roof but their LDL is low, particles are low, HDL is high, etc., their absolute risk is pretty low. The presence of high Lp(a) multiplies that risk by a factor. But multiplying a small number by a factor still leaves you with a small number. The same is true for LDL particles. Thus the target for treatment depends on the individual's overall risk profile."

– Dr. Ronald Krauss

Once again, nutrition rather than drugs constitutes the best therapy. Furthermore, when Lp(a) numbers start to tumble, so do other risk markers—it's a ripple effect that cannot be ignored. "As your Lp(a) number starts to come down, all your other lipid markers tend to become laughably excellent," said Dr. Davis. "In other words, HDL cholesterol can reach 80, 90, 110. We're talking about the elimination of small LDL particles—down to zero—and triglyceride levels of 30. Also, fasting blood glucose values in the 80s and hemoglobin A1c levels in the 4–5 range. Many Americans are currently prediabetic on their way to becoming diabetic. C-reactive protein can reach zero. If we reduced Lp(a) to zero but caused all sorts of problems in the process—well, doing that would be stupid."

6. High-Sensitivity C-Reactive Protein (hs-CRP)

MOMENT OF CLARITY: "There are good markers you can look at, such as high-sensitivity CRP, that tell you if you have oxidative stress. You don't really need the fancy tests for that."

– Dr. Fred Pescatore

High-sensitivity C-reactive protein (hs-CRP) is found in the blood and measures the state of inflammation in the body. This is the primary marker of inflammation and, therefore, the primary marker determining the overall health of your arteries. The higher your levels of CRP, the greater your risk of developing heart disease—and that's even if the rest of your cholesterol numbers look amazing.

Cholesterol has been vilified as the culprit in heart disease, but the case should be made (as we did in chapter 2) for inflammation, which is a much more serious problem than most people even realize. The higher your CRP levels, the greater your risk of heart disease. Healthy levels are between 0 and 3.0 mg/dL, with the ideal hs-CRP below 1. Reducing sugars, grains, and vegetable oils in your diet is the most effective way of reducing inflammation in your body.

7. Oral Glucose Tolerance Test (OGTT) and Fasting Blood Sugar Test

MOMENT OF CLARITY: "Don't check your cholesterol. Test your blood sugar."

– Dr. Donald Miller

This book is all about cholesterol, so what does your blood sugar response have to do with heart health? Turns out that as blood sugar and insulin go (that is, how well you are able to manage your blood sugar and insulin levels before and after meals), so goes your risk of both diabetes *and* heart disease. Dr. Patel frequently runs an oral glucose tolerance test (OGTT) and fasting blood sugar on his patients.

"My workhorse for determining insulin resistance is a two-hour glucose tolerance test," Dr. Patel said. "A study has shown that the one-hour post-prandial [after eating] blood glucose level is most predictive of becoming diabetic over the next eight years. If that one-hour number is greater than 150, you are thirteen times more likely to become diabetic in the next eight years, regardless of whether your fasting or two-hour blood sugar numbers are normal. So you could have completely normal fasting levels of 85 and a completely normal two-hour level of 115. But if your one-hour level is 150 or higher, you're still at risk. What this means is you can catch diabetes very early on by looking at this one-hour postprandial blood sugar. As a result, we can catch insulin resistance twenty to twenty-five years before a patient would develop diabetes."

MOMENT OF CLARITY: "Chronic overconsumption of carbohydrates causes chronic spikes in blood glucose and insulin. So if you have chronically high levels of insulin, then you're likely synthesizing more LDL cholesterol. High-carbohydrate diets negatively influence lipid metabolism and inflammatory processes. This proinflammatory state is the precursor to heart disease, neurodegenerative diseases, and even cancer. What carbohydrate restriction corrects are these postprandial spikes in the blood glucose. Large spikes in blood glucose can activate proinflammatory genes that drive pathological processes. Postprandial glucose spikes are especially dangerous for older folks, who are more likely to be sedentary and at risk of age-related cognitive decline."

— Dr. Dominic D'Agostino

The OGTT requires that you fast for eight to twelve hours. At that point, blood is drawn to test your fasting level of blood sugar and insulin. Then you are given a liquid containing 75 g of glucose and your blood is rechecked at thirty- and sixty-minute intervals for the duration of the test. It can be as short as two hours or as long as five. (I've done the five-hour version, and it's no fun, but it provides invaluable information.) "Some people complain about the two-hour glucose tolerance test," said Dr. Patel. "But not after I find abnormal results and the patient who thought he was healthy finds out he's not. It helps us to make the appropriate changes to make him better."

"So I think fasting insulin levels or perhaps insulin levels one hour after a glucose tolerance test are important. That's where you are getting to the heart of the issue in cardio-metabolic health."

– Dr. Malcolm Kendrick

Dr. Cate Shanahan regularly tests for insulin resistance in her patients because it "is the first measurable sign of the metabolic derangements that lead to heart attacks and strokes." But even before the test, she asks questions. "It's old-fashioned history taking," she said. "I ask patients whether or not they feel any of the symptoms of hypoglycemia, such as low energy or a weak, tired feeling, as if they needed to eat ASAP. That near-emergency feeling is not simple hunger; it's what happens when you can't easily access your energy stores. If your body can't burn fat, then you feel terrible when your blood sugar levels start to drop. Suddenly there's no energy! What are you going to do? Your body goes into panic mode, releasing adrenaline and other hormones so that the liver digs deeper into its own glycogen supply. Those hormones can make you feel edgy, nauseated, weak, shaky, and irritable. Getting that 'hypoglycemic' feeling between meals is a powerful warning. Don't ignore it. Whenever I hear that, I almost always see something wrong in one or more of the six metabolic snapshot lab tests—triglycerides, HDL, fasting blood glucose, A1c, white blood cells, and red blood cells."

Dr. Shanahan told me that a fasting blood sugar level above 92 indicates "other problems going on." I've often said that one of the best at-home medical devices you can own is a glucometer, which tests blood sugar levels. They are sold at any pharmacy or Walmart, and with just a few finger pricks before and after meals, you can see exactly how that slice of pizza or banana-nut muffin is really impacting your blood sugar levels (here's a hint: it ain't pretty!). You'll learn very quickly which foods spike your blood sugar, leading to hunger and changes in your mood, and which ones keep you nice and steady, with full hunger control and a general state of well-being. Ahhhhhh.

8. Apolipoprotein E (ApoE)

Since Apolipoprotein E, or ApoE, is inherited from your parents, you only need to test for it once in your life. There is no ideal range, but your number can tell you whether you are susceptible to a number of diseases, including cardiovascular illnesses. It can also help you to determine the diet and lifestyle that is best for you.

Science is still emerging on the ApoE genotype, and once again Dr. Davis is at the cutting-edge of the research into this. "We are living in the dawn of this age where we now have this whole collection of new genetic markers, most of which we have no idea what to do with," he explained. "ApoE is just one collection of these recognition proteins that give some insight into how people respond to diet. Everybody has two ApoE genes— one from Mom and one from Dad—and there are only 2, 3, and 4, so you can be a 2/2, 2/3, 3/3, 3/4, or 4/4. About 60 percent of the population has 3/3, so that is the most common ApoE number."

I happen to have an ApoE genotype of 3/3, which I've learned is a great number and the most common in the population. People who are a 3/4 or 4/4 are in the danger zone. "People with ApoE 4/4 tend to have a lot of problems with heart disease because of exaggerated lipoprotein abnormalities," said Dr. Davis. "But these people are very uncommon—less than 1 percent of the total population."

And what if you are among the 25 percent of the population who have at least one ApoE 4 gene? "Many people with the ApoE 4 genotype are very sensitive to fats," Dr. Davis said. "Unfortunately, it causes a lot of my cardiologist colleagues to say having ApoE 4 means you should follow a low-fat diet. That's ridiculous! If you have ApoE 4 and you follow a low-fat diet, you can become just as diabetic and fat as anybody else because a low-fat diet by definition is a high-carbohydrate diet. It's wrong to say that people with ApoE 4 have to eliminate fats; they simply need to figure out the optimal amount."

Once again, it all comes down to carbohydrates. "The first order of business with somebody with ApoE 4 is to cut your carbs," Dr. Davis said. "It's no different from anyone else because this can still be a culprit in your health. See how it plays out with your small LDL and think about further cutting carbohydrates if the numbers aren't where you need them to be."

It can be helpful if we look at this through the prism of our early ancestors. "Anthropologists have the very interesting, if badly named, 'thrifty gene' hypothesis," Dr. Davis explained. "This is the idea that there are genetic variants that prepare humans for periods of deprivation. For instance, 73,000 years ago there was an enormous volcanic eruption on the island of Sumatra in Indonesia. When the volcano erupted, it sent twenty-six cubic miles of mountain into the air, causing a six-year-long cooling trend: Dust hid the sun, causing the worldwide temperature to drop twenty-five degrees. Plants died, animals died, and humans died—only a few thousand remained. These people had to survive by scratching out a living in the barest of circumstances. The ones who survived were the best suited—the strongest, the ones who were most adapted to deprivation. Those few thousand people were the ancestors of all seven billion of the humans on earth today. That means we inherited genetic patterns that are adaptive to times of deprivation. I believe it could be argued that ApoE variance are just those kind of 'thrifty genes.'"

Dr. Davis noted that those with the ApoE 4 gene are particularly "well-suited to deprivation" through regular periods of intermittent fasting, especially since they are so sensitive to fat. "Nobody wants to give up eating for three days and then feast on the organs of a wild boar while scratching out a few leaves, nuts, and mushrooms in between," said Dr. Davis. "Now we're faced with this world of plenty, an unending flow of food—what for some with the ApoE 4 genotype is an excess for the genetic handling of fats. They should start by cutting back on fats a little, see how they react, and then go for a little more."

For those with the Apo4 gene unwilling to make such sacrifices—well, this could be one of those times when a drug would be recommended. "We could argue that because people don't want to feel deprived and live like our ancestors, maybe this is one of those situations where statins might be helpful," said Dr. Davis. "I don't ever want to hear people say that I think everyone should take statins because that's absurd! Statins are abused and misused by the medical profession. But I think in the same way we use antibiotics for infections, there are situations where statins do provide a legitimate benefit, especially for someone with an ApoE 4 genotype. But, as I said, that would never be my first strategy."

Some people may become discouraged when they test their ApoE genotype and realize they have a 4 in their results. Dr. Davis tells them to cheer up because he believes this is more of a blessing than a curse. "I remind patients frequently that if you have one of these 'thrifty gene' issues, you don't have a problem but a gift from our ancestors. It may not feel that way, but you have the advantage of being better prepared for deprivation and survival. So it is in some ways a blessing to have these things. Unfortunately, it doesn't seem that way in a world of plenty where we have access to essentially unlimited quantities of food."

What about people who have ApoE 2? Are there any special dietary considerations for them? Absolutely—and here comes that broken record again! According to Davis, "If you have one ApoE 2 gene, you have an incredible sensitivity to carbohydrates. This is because carbohydrate-triggered lipoproteins persist for an uncommonly long time, making liver receptor function about 99 percent less effective. So if you eat something made of grains or sugars, the lipoproteins persist in the bloodstream for prolonged periods, up to several weeks. But in a world of deprivation, that may have served you well because you had these lipoproteins to give you energy over an extended period. However, if you are an ApoE 2/2, it can cause a very exaggerated pattern, like very high triglycerides, thereby reducing HDL and expression of small LDL particles. So, from a heart disease standpoint, this has some serious implications. These people are also prone to diabetes."

As you can see, knowing your ApoE genotype can provide a lot of nutrition and lifestyle guidance. "Understanding genetic markers helps you understand why a hundred people all doing the same exact thing in diet and lifestyle will have a hundred different responses," Dr. Davis said.

Not everyone is a fan of this ApoE testing. "It is worthless with regard to heart disease," said Dr. Krauss. "It is much more strongly related to Alzheimer's disease than heart disease and this information has to be used with great care. To base any decisions, either diagnostic or therapeutic, for reducing heart disease risk based on this test is misguided—it's an awful lot about very little. It's hard to justify an expensive test like that without any evidence that having the result makes a difference in the outcome of treatment. Focusing on ApoE right now is like picking low-hanging fruit but leaving 98 percent on the tree."

ApoE genotype testing costs between $100 and $500. Obviously, only you can determine whether that one-time cost is worth what the test reveals.

In the next chapter, we'll put all your newfound knowledge to the test. *Awww man, I didn't know there was gonna be a test!* Don't worry; I'm pretty sure you'll ace it, now that you know exactly what the HDL is wrong (or not) with your numbers.

DOCTOR'S NOTE FROM DR. ERIC WESTMAN: Medicine is
practiced in many different ways across the country and
around the world, depending on when and where your
doctor was trained. So it should come as no surprise that
much of the information in this book will be brand-new to
your doctor.

KEY CHOLESTEROL CLARITY CONCEPTS

→ **ApoB is a cheap and widely available test to assess cardiovascular risk.**

→ **Testing for LDL-P gives you the total number of LDL particles in your blood.**

→ **Small LDL-P are the dense, atherogenic LDL particles you want to eliminate.**

→ **Non-HDL cholesterol is a newer way to calculate your heart-health risk.**

→ **Lipoprotein(a) is a genetic cardiovascular risk marker that needs to be lowered.**

→ **High-sensitivity C-reactive protein is the primary test to determine inflammation.**

→ **A glucose tolerance test and a fasting blood sugar test assess insulin resistance.**

→ **ApoE genotype testing can tell you the best kind of eating regimen for your particular body type.**

Chapter 21 ——————

Test Your Ability to Read Cholesterol Test Results

MOMENT OF CLARITY: "We have what I regard as a form of brainwashing that has gone on for the last few decades around cholesterol. Some of this has come from people who mean well but have maybe been misguided."

— Dr. John Briffa

MOMENT OF CLARITY: "Ultimately, all of this is in the hands of patients educating themselves about this."

— Dr. Cate Shanahan

Since I first started writing about the subject of cholesterol on my blog many years ago, hundreds of readers have e-mailed me their cholesterol test results and asked me to tell them what they mean. While I am certainly no doctor, I am happy to offer my layperson's opinion based on the collective wisdom of people like the experts I have featured in this book. It can be tricky to attempt to make an assessment about health based on the numbers on a blood test, but hopefully, by this point, you understand a whole lot more about the various markers and what really matters most. (And just in case you missed it, that would *not* be your LDL and total cholesterol.)

So let's take the information in this book and give it some practical application. The following are thirty real-life examples of actual cholesterol test results. Your mission (if you choose to accept it) is to interpret them based on everything you've learned. See if you can identify those with healthy results, those who could stand to improve their numbers, and those who have poor health risk markers. Ready? Here we go!

EXAMPLE 1: Female with family history of heart disease

LDL-P	889
Lipids LDL-C	88
HDL-C	62
Triglycerides	44
Cholesterol, Total	159
Small LDL-P	104
LP-IR Score	9

Healthy, work needed, or poor markers? _____

EXAMPLE 2: Female taking medication for high blood pressure

LDL-P	2000
LDL-C	146
HDL-C	60
Triglycerides	76
Cholesterol, Total	221
Small LDL-P	1188
LP-IR Score	60

Healthy, work needed, or poor markers? _____

EXAMPLE 3: Female taking 15 mg of statin drug therapy

Total Cholesterol	222
LDL-C	119
HDL-C	73
Triglycerides	148
LDL-P	2171
Small LDL-P	972

Healthy, work needed, or poor markers? _____

EXAMPLE 4: Female off statin drug therapy for six months

Cholesterol, Total	299
HDL-C	88
LP-IR Score	4
LDL-C	199
LDL-P	2202
Small LDL-P	179
Triglycerides	61
VLDL Size	Too small to measure

Healthy, work needed, or poor markers? _____

EXAMPLE 5: Male whose doctor recommends Lipitor/fish oil

LDL-P	2228
LDL-C	112
HDL-C	48
Triglycerides	233
Cholesterol, Total	207
Small LDL-P	1580
LP-IR Score	51

Healthy, work needed, or poor markers? _____

EXAMPLE 6: Female on 10mg Simvastatin

Cholesterol, Total	209
LDL-C	101
HDL-C	72
Triglycerides	115
Apo B	100
LDL-P	1206
Small LDL-P	446
Lp(a)	15

Healthy, work needed. or poor markers? _____

EXAMPLE 7: Female, 42, who suffered a heart attack and is on a statin drug

Total cholesterol	134
Triglycerides	58
HDL-C	58
LDL-C	73
VLDL	12
LDL-P	1239
Small LDL-P	600
Lp(a)	3.9
C-Reactive Protein	.3

Healthy, work needed, or poor markers? _____

EXAMPLE 8: Female refusing to take a statin drug

Total Cholesterol	253
LDL-C	174
HDL-C	58
Triglycerides	106
LDL-P	2546
Small LDL-P	626

Healthy, work needed, or poor markers? _____

EXAMPLE 9: Female Type II diabetic with high blood pressure

LDL-P	2459
LDL-C	172
HDL	51
Triglycerides	280
Cholesterol, Total	279
Small LDL-P	1181

Healthy, work needed, or poor markers? _____

EXAMPLE 10: Male weight-lifter, muscular build

LDL-P	1248
Small LDL-P	413
HDL-C	55
Triglycerides	43
LP-IR Score	22
C-Reactive Protein	.32

Healthy, work needed, or poor markers? _____

EXAMPLE 11: Female on wheat-free Paleo diet

Total Cholesterol	278
LDL-C	192
HDL-C	78
Triglycerides	42
VLDL	Too small to measure
LP-IR Score	5
LDL-P	1602
Small LDL-P	113

Healthy, work needed, or poor markers? _____

EXAMPLE 12: MaleType 2 diabetic taking Metformin

Total Cholesterol	187
LDL-C	130
HDL-C	46
Triglycerides	57
LDL-P	1746
Small LDL-P	834
LP-IR Score	30

Healthy, work needed, or poor markers? _____

EXAMPLE 13: Female athlete with family history of heart disease

Total Cholesterol	357
LDL-C	289
HDL-C	55
Triglycerides	66
LDL-P	2001
Small LDL-P	131

Healthy, work needed, or poor markers? _____

EXAMPLE 14: Male whose doctor insists on statin drug therapy

LDL-P	1495
LDL-C	108
HDL-C	54
Triglycerides	65
Total Cholesterol	175
Small LDL-P	690

Healthy, work needed, or poor markers? _____

EXAMPLE #15: Female told by doctor that she'll have a heart attack

Total cholesterol	309
HDL-C	69
LDL-C	232
Triglycerides	42
LDL-P	2505
Small LDL-P	852
LP-IR Score	10

Healthy, work needed or poor markers? _____

EXAMPLE 16: Female senior citizen taking Lipitor

Total Cholesterol	189
LDL-P	1995
LDL-C	111
HDL-C	45
Triglycerides	166
Small LDL-P	1485
LP-IR Score	75

Healthy, work needed, or poor markers? _____

EXAMPLE 17: Female on low-carb, high-fat diet

Total Cholesterol	303
LDL-C	189
HDL-C	103
Triglycerides	53
LDL-P	1476
Small LDL-P	104
LP-IR Score	1

Healthy, work needed, or poor markers? _____

EXAMPLE 18: Male with family history of heart disease and diabetes

LDL-P	1133
LDL-C	117
HDL-C	61
Triglycerides	39
Total Cholesterol	186
SMALL LDL-P	90
VLDL	Too small to measure
LP-IR Score	4

Healthy, work needed, or poor markers? _____

EXAMPLE 19: Male eating high-carb, low-fat diet

Total Cholesterol	128
LDL-C	45
HDL-C	27
Triglycerides	351
LDL-P	1146
Small LDL-P	1077
LP-IR Score	46
Apo B	68
C-Reactive Protein	1.2
ApoE Genotype	¾

Healthy, work needed, or poor markers? _____

EXAMPLE 20: Female eating a low-carb, high-fat diet

Total Cholesterol	418
LDL-C	305
HDL-C	104
VLDL	11
Triglycerides	56

Healthy, work needed, or poor markers? _____

EXAMPLE 21: Male eating low-carb, high-fat diet

LDL-P	1924
LDL-C	152
HDL-C	59
Triglycerides	46
Total Cholesterol	220
Small LDL-P	625
LP-IR Score	18

Healthy, work needed, or poor markers? _____

EXAMPLE 22: Male actively lowering stress, eating low-carb diet

Total Cholesterol	201
LDL-C	127
HDL-C	67
Triglycerides	33
LDL-P	1348
Small LDL-P	137
LP-IR Score	13

Healthy, work needed, or poor markers? _____

EXAMPLE 23: Female on blood pressure medication

Total Cholesterol	220
LDL-C	106
HDL	50
Triglycerides	320
LDL-P	1890
Small LDL-P	1073

Healthy, work needed, or poor markers? _____

EXAMPLE 24: Male wondering if he needs cholesterol drugs

Total Cholesterol	210
LDL-C	146
HDL-C	45
Triglycerides	95
LDL-P	1709
Small LDL-P	619
LP-IR Score	35

Healthy, work needed, or poor markers? _____

EXAMPLE 25: Female on low-carb, high-fat Primal diet

Total cholesterol	269
LDL-P	1829
LDL-C	182
HDL-C	77
Triglycerides	50
Small LDL-P	146
C-Reactive Protein	.58
LP-IR Score	4

Healthy, work needed, or poor markers? _____

EXAMPLE 26: Female who wants to avoid taking statins

Total Cholesterol	278
LDL-C	200
HDL-C	51
Triglycerides	137
LDL-P	2049
Small LDL-P	627

Healthy, work needed, or poor markers? _____

EXAMPLE 27: Female on high-fat, low-carb diet

Total Cholesterol	250
LDL-C	168
HDL-C	69
Triglycerides	64
LDL-P	1699
Small LDL-P	104

Healthy, work needed, or poor markers? _____

EXAMPLE 28: Female on high-fat, low-carb diet

Total Cholesterol	193
LDL-C	105
HDL-C	81
Triglycerides	36
LDL-P	934
Small LDL-P	90

Healthy, work needed, or poor markers? _____

EXAMPLE 29: Female Type 2 diabetic on low-carb diet

Total Cholesterol	216
LDL-C	132
HDL-C	74
Triglycerides	51
LDL-P	1524
Small LDL-P	166
LP-IR Score	12

Healthy, work needed, or poor markers? _____

EXAMPLE 30: Male who lost over 180 pounds on a low-carb diet

Total Cholesterol	359
LDL-C	285
HDL-C	65
Triglycerides	46
VLDL	12
C-Reaction Protein	0.55
LDL-P	3451
Small LDL-P	221
ApoB	238

Healthy, work needed, or poor markers? _____

That last example is my NMR Lipoprofile cholesterol test results, which were run in October 2012. Most conventional doctors would look at my total cholesterol and LDL-C and immediately want to put me on a high-dose statin drug. But from what we've learned about cholesterol numbers, that's not the whole story, is it? Take a look at the markers that matter. My HDL-C level of 65 indicates outstanding heart health. My triglycerides, at 46, are well within range of stellar. My VLDL of 12 is microscopically low (a good thing!), and my C-reactive protein shows nearly zero inflammation at just 0.55. While my LDL-P is indeed very high at 3,451 (and the parallel marker of ApoB is also very high at 238), just 6 percent of those particles are the small, dense, bad kind—which means 94 percent are the large, fluffy, good kind you want to have. That's not bad for a guy who used to weigh over four hundred pounds and used to pop cholesterol-lowering prescription drugs like Tic-Tacs!

So how did you do on the test? While, as you now know, it's impossible to simply look at cholesterol numbers and make a full assessment of people's health, you can certainly extrapolate the general state of their heart health, based on these numbers. Here's the ranking based on everything you've learned:

Healthy markers—1, 4, 7, 10, 11, 13, 14, 15, 17, 18, 20, 22, 25, 27, 28, 29, 30
Some work needed—2, 3, 6, 8, 12, 21, 24, 26
Poor markers—5, 9, 16, 19, 23

Isn't it interesting that despite the statin drug therapy used by patients 3, 6, and 16, they all have excellent LDL-C and poor triglyceride as well as Small LDL-P numbers? Interesting, but I hope not surprising at this point.

KEY CHOLESTEROL CLARITY CONCEPTS

→ **Analyzing cholesterol blood test results can be tricky business.**

→ **Distinguishing healthy cholesterol panels from unhealthy ones should be easier now.**

Epilogue ————————————————————

Now That You've Been Enlightened, What Happens Next?

MOMENT OF CLARITY: "We talk about this issue to anyone who will listen. It's a very hard, uphill climb, but we're getting more and more people to start paying attention."

— Dr. Jonny Bowden

I have received such an enormous gift—the gift of health—and I owe it all to doing virtually the opposite of what conventional health experts had been telling me for years. Weight loss is one thing, but getting your health in order is so much more rewarding, especially when you yourself have done the work to achieve it. How many of your own friends, coworkers, and family members are simply following orders from their doctors about how to be healthy? And it's all dead wrong!

MOMENT OF CLARITY: "There is a group of patients who are going to question what they have been told about cholesterol. They are going to be willing to go there to see what works and what doesn't work. Ultimately, even more people are going to have to be motivated in order to make those kinds of changes happen. That motivation may come from someone having a side effect from taking statins or the fear of having a complication that might occur from taking the drug. The biggest motivator is the fact that someone is not getting the desired results. This is when people are open to an alternate pathway and an alternative treatment program to the statin medications."

— Dr. Philip Blair

MOMENT OF CLARITY: "The truth is saturated fat and dietary cholesterol have never been shown to cause heart disease. People are shocked and question why they have been taught to believe just the opposite. Your heart really needs good fats from salmon, egg yolks, avocados, nuts, seeds, olive oil, coconut oil, and (gasp!) even butter. And when you look at some of the detrimental effects that come from eating grains and refined foods, I try to make them understand so it will make sense to them. A big part of this is having people just try this. If you don't believe me, try it. It comes down to how people feel and whether they can make it through their workday with enough energy to come home and play with their kids. When that part starts working for them, people will be more willing to embrace this."

– Cassie Bjork

Writing this book has been one of the most gratifying experiences of my entire life and it's a book I've been wanting to write for years. Now more than ever, this information needs to be shared with as many people as possible to save them from going down the inevitable road of health destruction under the guise of obtaining health. It is my sincere hope that this book has in some small way encouraged you to rethink everything you once believed was true about cholesterol, nutrition, and health. If that has happened, then I consider my mission accomplished. I'd love to hear your story about the impact this book has made on your thinking regarding cholesterol via e-mail at livinlowcarbman@charter.net. Breaking down the walls of what we've always believed to be fact is incredibly challenging, but it is not impossible. As more and more people become clear about cholesterol, a major paradigm shift will take place and the veil of ignorance will be lifted.

MOMENT OF CLARITY: "A few years ago, I as a doctor had all the knowledge. If you wanted some knowledge, you came to me and you could get it. Nowadays, you can do a few clicks on your computer and get information, and maybe I can get some knowledge out of that. Information is no longer the doctor's exclusive purview. It's now available to everybody."

– Dr. Dwight Lundell

MOMENT OF CLARITY: "Doctors who are busy and don't read a lot of things have been misled into thinking that cholesterol is what you've got to look at. And that's wrong!"

– Dr. Donald Miller

MOMENT OF CLARITY: "Yes, you do have a lot of control over these things, if you're given the right information."

– Dr. William Davis

MOMENT OF CLARITY: "We do so many artificial things in this world. It's like a dog chasing its own tail. We do so many bad things to ourselves and then treat those things with drugs that we think we need to have. Then we do something else that's bad for our body and then we follow it up with something else. It's just a spiral that never ends."

– Dr. Fred Pescatore

I encourage you to share this book and what you've learned with everyone you know and love. And don't stop there: We've only just scratched the surface! Empower yourself with even more knowledge by continuing the education process, and become your own best health advocate. By eating and living in the ways discussed in this book, you not only benefit personally, but you also become a living example of what it means to be truly, naturally heart healthy. Who knows? Your doctor might even learn a thing or two by seeing your example. Change happens one step, one person, at a time.

So what are you waiting for? Let's change the world!

MOMENT OF CLARITY: "I feel as if I'm an old-fashioned doctor. I don't need a blood test to figure out what's going on in someone's body and what to do about it. I use blood tests for patients to see their progress."

– Dr. Cate Shanahan

MOMENT OF CLARITY: "Every day more and more people are understanding that it's not the cholesterol that's the problem, but the particles carrying the cholesterol. And they're buying into this idea that a high-fat diet can be healthy for them because of the beneficial effect, among many other things, on the LDL particle size and number."

– Gary Taubes

DOCTOR'S NOTE FROM DR. ERIC WESTMAN: Because of all the vested interests—food and pharmaceutical companies and the "guild" of doctors—the best advice I can give you is to follow your own health markers, educate yourself, and then try something to see how this affects your health.

Jimmy Moore's Cholesterol Test Results from 2008 to 2013

DATE	LDL-P	LDL-C	HDL-C	Triglycerides	Total Cholesterol	Small LDL-P	VLDL
4/18/13	2730	236	66	38	310	478	7
2/28/13	N/A	309	77	72	400	N/A	14
12/14/12	N/A	332	75	60	419	N/A	12
10/25/12	3451	285	65	46	359	221	9
4/25/12	N/A	257	67	88	342	N/A	17
2/28/12	N/A	290	78	89	386	N/A	18
10/20/09	2130	278	57	79	351	535	16
7/13/09	2091	228	60	49	298	1261	10
5/5/08	1453	250	65	86	332	300	17
5/5/08	N/A	246	65	77	326	N/A	15

Cholesterol Conversion Chart
mg/dL to mmol/L

mg/dL	mmol/L	mg/dL	mmol/L
2-30	.1-.8	80	2.1
3	.1	85	2.2
5	.1	90	2.3
10	.3	92	2.4
12	.3	97	2.5
14	.4	98	2.5
23	.6	100	2.6
25	.6	100-129	2.6-3.3
30	.8	101	2.6
32	.8	105	2.7
40	1	110	2.8
40-49	1-1.3	112	2.9
41	1.1	115	3
42	1.1	127	3.3
43	1.1	130	3.4
50	1.3	130-159	3.4-4.1
50-59	1.3-1.5	138	3.6
52	1.3	139	3.6
53	1.4	140	3.6
58	1.5	145	3.8
60	1.6	147	3.8
65	1.7	148	3.8
70	1.8	150	3.9
71	1.8	150-199	3.9-5.1
72	1.9	154	4
78	2	155	4

mg/dL	mmol/L	mg/dL	mmol/L
157	4.1	227	5.9
160	4.1	230	5.9
160-189	4.1-4.9	232	6
160-240	4.1-6.2	234	6.1
164	4.2	236	6.1
165	4.3	238	6.2
180	4.7	240	6.2
181	4.7	245	6.3
185	4.8	246	6.4
190	4.9	250	6.5
193	5	251	6.5
195-225	5-5.8	252	6.5
199	5.1	255	6.6
200	5.2	263	6.8
200-239	5.2-6.2	268	6.9
200-499	5.2-12.9	270	7
201	5.2	280	7.2
203	5.3	300	7.8
204	5.3	310	8
210	5.4	322	8.3
215	5.6	350	9.1
217	5.6	400	10.3
220	5.7	500	12.9
222	5.7	509	13.2
223	5.8	680	17.6
225	5.8		

Triglyceride Conversion Chart
mg/dL to mmol/L

mg/dL	mmol/L	mg/dL	mmol/L
30	.3	95	1.1
33	.4	97	1.1
36	.4	98	1.1
39	.4	100	1.1
41	.5	106	1.2
42	.5	115	1.3
43	.5	130	1.5
44	.5	137	1.5
46	.5	148	1.7
50	.6	150	1.7
51	.6	154	1.7
52	.6	166	1.9
53	.6	199	2.2
56	.6	200	2.3
57	.6	227	2.6
58	.7	233	2.6
60	.7	280	3.2
61	.7	300	3.4
64	.7	320	3.6
65	.7	351	4
66	.7	499	5.6
70	.8	500	5.6
76	.9	800	9
80	.9		

Pounds to Kilograms

pound	kilogram	pound	kilogram
8	3.6	103	46.7
25	11.3	140	63.5
50	22.67	180	81.6
70	31.7	230	104.3
95	43	400	181.4
100	45.3	410	185.9

Cholesterol Clarity Testing Guide with Optimal Ranges

Standard Lipid Panel	
Total Cholesterol	Mostly irrelevant, but women should be 250 mg/dL or below and men should be 220 mg/dL or below
LDL-C	130 mg/dL or below, but higher levels are not necessarily relevant to your heart health risk.
HDL-C	Above 50mg/dL is good, but 70 mg/dL or higher is best
VLDL-C	Between 10 and 14 mg/dL
Triglycerides	100 mg/dL or below, but under 70mg/dL is best
Non-HDL Cholesterol	No evidence of an optimal level

Advanced Lipid Panel	
LDL-P	Below 1000 nmol/L, but unknown for people eating a high-fat, low-carb diet
Small LDL-P	20 percent or less of your LDL-P number and optimally less than 200 nmol/L
Lipoprotein(a)	A genetic marker with no standard methodology for measuring, the ranges will vary widely

Other Tests To Consider	
Apolipoprotein B (ApoB)	Parallel marker to LDL-P
Apolipoprotein E (ApoE) Genotype (one-time only test)	There is no ideal range, but test it once to know your genetic predisposition (3/3 is the most common and best number; 2/2, 3/4 and 4/4 are the worst)
High Sensitivity C-Reactive Protein (hs-CRP)	Between 0 and 3.0 mg/dL, with the ideal below 1
Fasting blood sugar	92 mg/dL or below
Oral glucose tolerance test (OGTT)	One-hour blood sugar reading under 150 mg/dL

Tests To Run If You Are Worried About High Cholesterol	
CT Heart Scan Calcium Score	An inexpensive, 3-minute test that measures for calcified plaque in your chest. The score you want is 0
Carotid Intima Media Thickness (IMT)	Measures the thickness of your arterial walls an early indicator of cardiovascular disease
Metametrix GI Effects stool test	Measures for any microscopic bugs in your intestines that could be wreaking havoc on your body

Recommended Resources

Books

Bowden, Dr. Jonny, and Dr. Stephen Sinatra. *The Great Cholesterol Myth: Why Lowering Your Cholesterol Won't Prevent Heart Disease—and the Statin-Free Plan That Will.* (2012)

Curtis, Dr. Ernest. *The Cholesterol Delusion.* (2010)

Ellison, Shane. *Hidden Truth about Cholesterol-Lowering Drugs.* (2005)

Enig, Dr. Mary. *Know Your Fats: The Complete Primer for Understanding the Nutrition of Fats, Oils and Cholesterol.* (2000)

Evans, David. *Cholesterol and Saturated Fat Prevent Heart Disease: Evidence from 101 Scientific Papers.* (2012)

Graveline, Dr. Duane. *Lipitor: Thief Of Memory.* (2006)

Graveline, Dr. Duane. *Statin Drugs Side Effects and the Misguided War on Cholesterol.* (2008)

Graveline, Dr. Duane, with Dr. Malcolm Kendrick. *The Statin Damage Crisis.* (2012)

Kendrick, Dr. Malcolm. *The Great Cholesterol Con: The Truth about What Really Causes Heart Disease and How to Avoid It.* (2008)

Kummerow, Dr. Fred. *Cholesterol Won't Kill You, But Trans Fat Could: Separating Scientific Fact from Nutritional Fiction in What You Eat.* (2008)

Ravnskov, Dr. Uffe. *The Cholesterol Myths: Exposing the Fallacy That Saturated Fat and Cholesterol Cause Heart Disease.* (2000)

Ravnskov, Dr. Uffe. *Fat and Cholesterol are Good for You.* (2009)

Ravnskov, Dr. Uffe. *Ignore the Awkward: How the Cholesterol Myths Are Kept Alive.* (2010)

Taubes, Gary. *Good Calories, Bad Calories: Fats, Carbs, and the Controversial Science of Diet and Health.* (2008)

Blogs

Dr. Peter Attia, http://www.eatingacademy.com

Dr. Chris Masterjohn, http://blog.cholesterol-and-health.com

Chris Kresser, http://chriskresser.com

Dr. Mark Hyman, http://drhyman.com

Dr. Barry Groves, http://www.second-opinions.co.uk

Dr. John Briffa, http://www.drbriffa.com

Dr. William Davis, http://www.wheatbellyblog.com

Dr. Malcolm Kendrick, http://www.drmalcolmkendrick.org

Dr. Stephen Sinatra, http://www.drsinatra.com

Dr. Jonny Bowden, http://www.jonnybowdenblog.com

Dr. Duane Graveline, http://www.spacedoc.com

Podcasts

The Livin' La Vida Low-Carb Show, http://www.thelivinlowcarbshow.com

Ask The Low-Carb Experts, http://www.askthelowcarbexperts.com

Low-Carb Conversations With Jimmy Moore & Friends,
http://www.lowcarbconversations.com

Revolution Health Radio, http://chriskresser.com/category/podcasts

The Paleo Solution Podcast, http://www. robbwolf.com/podcast

The Underground Wellness Show,
http://www.blogtalkradio.com/undergroundwellness

The Bulletproof Executive,
http://www.bulletproofexec.com/category/podcasts

The People's Pharmacy, http://www.peoplespharmacy.com/radio-shows

The Balanced Bites Podcast, http://balancedbites.com/podcast

The Fat-Burning Man Show,
http://www.fatburningman.com/category/podcasts

Latest In Paleo, http://www.latestinpaleo.com/paleo-podcast

Dishing Up Nutrition, http://www.weightandwellness.com/radio-show

Relentless Roger And The Caveman Doctor,
http://www.cavemandoctor.com/category/podcasts

Documentaries

$TATIN NATION, http://www.statinnation.net

Fat Head, http://www.fathead-movie.com

Other Useful Websites

The International Network of Cholesterol Skeptics (THINCS), http://www.thincs.org

High Cholesterol Action Plan, http://highcholesterolplan.chriskresser.com

Find a Paleo/low-carb friendly doctor

List Of Low-Carb Doctors, http://lowcarbdoctors.blogspot.com

Primal Docs, http://primaldocs.com

Paleo Physicians Network, http://paleophysiciansnetwork.com

Glossary

ApoB: a molecule (apolipoprotein) that is found on blood cholesterol particles. ApoB100 is found on low-density lipoproteins that are made in the liver. ApoB48 is found on chylomicron particles that are made in the intestine.

ApoE Genotype: the hereditary type of apolipoprotein E that certain people produce. The ApoE4 genotype may signal a higher risk for particular diseases.

Atherogenic: leading to the development of atherosclerosis.

Atherosclerosis: the thickening and hardening of arteries due to inflammation and the depositing of cholesterol and triglycerides in the arterial wall. Atherosclerosis is a primary cause of stroke, heart attacks, and aneurysms.

ATP III Cholesterol Guidelines: a set of guidelines, created by the U.S. National Institutes of Health's National Heart, Lung and Blood Institute, that suggest goals for blood cholesterol levels for doctors to use in treating patients. (This is the third report of the Expert Panel on Detection, Evaluation, and Treatment of High Blood Cholesterol in Adults; the fourth report is due out in 2014.)

Big Pharma: a term used to describe large companies that develop, manufacture, and sell pharmaceuticals (medications).

Blood Sugar: a molecule that carries energy in the blood. Also known as blood glucose. If the blood sugar remains elevated throughout the day, this is known as diabetes.

Carbohydrate: a molecule consisting of carbon, oxygen, and hydrogen that provides energy to the body. Carbohydrates are found in dietary sugars and starches.

Cardiovascular Disease: a term that includes atherosclerosis of the heart or other blood vessels.

Cholesterol: a molecule that is used for many purposes in the human body, including bolstering cell membranes, making steroid hormones (cortisol, aldosterone, sex hormones), repairing nerves, making bile, and creating and metabolizing vitamin D.

Cholesterol-Heart Hypothesis: the theory stating that dietary fat leads to an increase in blood cholesterol, and this increase in blood cholesterol leads to atherosclerosis of the arteries of the heart (coronary artery disease), and heart attacks.

Clogged Artery: partial or complete blockage of an artery due to atherosclerosis.

CoQ10 (coenzyme Q10): an important molecule that is used in the production of energy in the body and is also an antioxidant.

C-Reactive Protein (CRP): a protein found in the blood that assists in the inflammatory response. Higher levels of CRP increase the risk of developing diabetes and cardiovascular disease.

CT Heart Scan: a noninvasive test that can detect the early onset of heart disease.

Dolichols: members of the isoprenoid family produced by the mevalonate pathway Long-chain unsaturated organic compounds that play an important role in glycoprotein synthesis. Statin drugs have been shown to disrupt the action of dolichols by altering the glycoproteins that are meant to protect the body from harm.

Endothelial: referring to the endothelium, a thin layer of cells on the inner lining of the blood vessel (artery or vein).

Familial Hypercholesterolemia: a hereditary tendency to have high levels of low-density lipoproteins in the blood. The most severe form, known as homozygous FH, is rare (affecting about 1 in a million people). The more common form, known as heterozygous FH, affects about 1 in 500.

Fat: a molecule used for energy in the body; the primary storage form of energy in the body.

Gut Microbiota: bacteria found in the intestines.

HDL-C (high-density lipoprotein): a particle in the blood that carries cholesterol from the arteries to the liver.

Heart Disease: any disease affecting the heart, but most commonly used to describe atherosclerosis of the arteries of the heart. The arteries of the heart are called coronary arteries.

Hemoglobin A1c (also known as HgA1c or glycated hemoglobin): glycated hemoglobin (hemoglobin is a molecule that carries oxygen in the red blood cells) is a type of hemoglobin that increases as the blood sugar increases. Because red blood cells last about three months, glycated hemoglobin reflects the blood sugar level for the previous three months.

Homocysteine: a molecule used to alter other molecules in the body. High levels may increase the risk of atherosclerosis.

hsCRP (high-sensitivity C-reactive protein): a test that can detect small amounts of C-reactive protein, a marker of inflammation, in the blood.

Hypercholesterolemia: Increased levels of blood cholesterol of any kind.

Inflammation: a response in the body to fight infection or repair an injury.

Insulin: a hormone secreted by the pancreas and put into the bloodstream in response to an increase in blood sugar or protein. It assists in the transfer of sugar (glucose) and protein into the cells.

Ketogenic Diet: a dietary regimen consisting mainly of protein and fat, which increases the level of ketones in the bloodstream. Ketones are molecules that carry energy.

Leptin: a hormone made by fat cells that reduces the appetite.

LDL-C (low-density lipoprotein): lipoproteins made by the liver that carry cholesterol and fat-soluble vitamins from the liver to the cells. Also refers to the amount of cholesterol carried in the low-density lipoprotein particles in the blood.

LDL-P (low-density lipoprotein cholesterol particles, aka LDL particles): a measurement of the number of LDL particles in the blood, as opposed to the measurement of the amount of cholesterol carried by the LDL-C.

LDL-R (low-density lipoprotein cholesterol receptor): a protein in the membrane of cells that recognizes the ApoB100 on LDL particles and helps LDL enter the cells.

Lipid Hypothesis: the theory that dietary fat leads to an increase in blood cholesterol, and this increase in blood cholesterol leads to atherosclerosis of the arteries of the heart (coronary artery disease), and heart attacks.

Lipid Panel: a blood test that typically measures total cholesterol, low-density lipoprotein cholesterol, high-density lipoprotein cholesterol, and triglycerides.

Lipoproteins: molecules in the blood that carry cholesterol, triglycerides, and fat-soluble substances throughout the bloodstream.

Lipoprotein(a): an inherited alteration of LDLs that increases one's risk of cardiovascular disease.

Low-Carb, High-Fat (LCHF): an eating regimen that focuses on consuming few carbohydrates, popularized in countries like Sweden.

Low Cholesterol: lower than normal levels of cholesterol in the blood.

Mitochondria: components of cells that generate energy for the cell.

Monounsaturated fatty acids: fatty acids that contain one double bond.

NMR Lipoprofile: a test that measures the amounts and sizes of blood cholesterol particles.

Non-HDL Cholesterol: the amount of cholesterol not on the HDL particles; determined by using a lipid panel.

Omega-3 fatty acids: molecules used by the body for structure and energy.

Omega-6 fatty acids: a molecule used by the body for structure and energy. Found in vegetable oils, these fatty acids are used to make molecules used in inflammation.

Oxidation: akin to the rusting of iron, oxidation in the body leads to aging and inflammation.

Paleo and Primal Diets: based on the notion that what humans ate as hunter-gatherers is healthiest, these are ways of eating that exclude processed foods and dairy products.

Pattern A: a pattern of blood cholesterol found in people with low levels of small LDL cholesterol.

Pattern B: a pattern of blood cholesterol found in people with high levels of small LDL cholesterol. People with this pattern have a greater risk of atherosclerosis.

Polyunsaturated Fat: fatty acids that have more than one double bond

Saturated Fat: fatty acids that have no double bonds.

Small LDL-P: thought to be "the bad guys," small LDL particles contribute to the process of atherosclerosis.

Statins: a group of drugs that block the production of cholesterol in the liver.

T3 and T4: the two forms of thyroid hormone that exist in the bloodstream. T4 is made in the thyroid gland and converted to T3 in the cells.

TGA and ALS: transient global amnesia (TGA) and amyotrophic lateral sclerosis (ALS), commonly referred to as Lou Gehrig's disease; both have been shown to be among the major neurodegenerative side effects of taking cholesterol-lowering statin drugs. Dr. Duane Graveline, one of this book's experts, has written extensively about this.

Thyroid Stimulating Hormone (TSH): a hormone made by the pituitary gland that signals the thyroid gland to make more thyroid hormone. High levels of TSH suggest that hypothyroidism may be present.

Total Cholesterol: a blood measurement of the amount of cholesterol carried on lipoprotein particles.

Total Cholesterol–to–HDL Cholesterol Ratio: dividing one's total choles-terol number by one's HDL cholesterol number; a higher ratio is associ-ated with a higher risk of atherosclerosis.

Triglyceride: a molecule used for energy in the body.

Triglycerides-to-HDL Ratio: dividing the triglycerides by the HDL; a higher ratio is associated with a higher risk of atherosclerosis.

Vegetable Oil: the major oils people use for cooking, including soybean, canola, sunflower, safflower, peanut, and cottonseed. Although these oils are marketed as "heart healthy," they are highly processed, proinflamma-tory, foodlike substances that are extremely high in omega-6 fatty acids, leading to oxidation of LDL cholesterol—the precursor to heart disease.

Vegetarian Diet: a way of eating that only derives nutrition from vegetable sources.

VLDL (very low-density lipoprotein): made in the liver, a VLDL particle is an LDL particle that contains triglycerides.

Index

Acknowledgments

Jimmy Moore: I'd like to thank a few key people instrumental in making this vitally important book a reality. To my wife, Christine, who put up with me spending many months on end leaving the house to go to the public library for hours at a time: I'm grateful for all her sacrifices of time away from her husband. (Now I can get back to kicking her tail in Wii Disc Golf again!) To my amazing coauthor, Dr. Eric Westman, who brought immeasurable wisdom, experience, and passion to this much-neglected topic. It was an honor to be partners with you in sharing this message, and I look forward to collaborating with you again on *Keto Clarity* in 2014. To all twenty-nine of my cholesterol experts, who so graciously shared their time and expertise through exclusive interviews I conducted with them on this subject: This book would not be the same without your invaluable "Moment of Clarity" quotes. To my publishing team—Erich, Michele, and everyone at Victory Belt: What an honor to be a part of the incredible, life-changing work you are doing through your books! Kudos to you for making this one of the most enjoyable and gratifying experiences of my entire life. And finally, to you, the reader: I want to acknowledge you because it's obvious you care about your own health and that of your loved ones—enough that you would take the time to read this book and think outside the box of conventional wisdom. The first steps in bringing about lasting change are education and implementation. Never stop learning and living it!

Dr. Eric Westman: I am grateful to the education provided by the Duke University data-driven mindset. I have learned through classwork on evidence-based medicine, conducting clinical research, and especially from the patients that I have had the good fortune to help as their doctor. Most of all, I am grateful to my family and friends for their support.